MW01291512

THE GIFT OF
HEALING
HANDS

A GUIDE

Thank you for sharing your gifts,

Marina Mangano D.C., RYT

Marina Mangano DC

BALBOA.PRESS
A DIVISION OF HAY HOUSE

Balboa Press books may be ordered through booksellers or by contacting:

Balboa Press
A Division of Hay House
1663 Liberty Drive
Bloomington, IN 47403
www.balboapress.com
844-682-1282

Because of the dynamic nature of the Internet, any web addresses or links contained in this book may have changed since publication and may no longer be valid. The views expressed in this work are solely those of the author and do not necessarily reflect the views of the publisher, and the publisher hereby disclaims any responsibility for them.

The author of this book does not dispense medical advice or prescribe the use of any technique as a form of treatment for physical, emotional, or medical problems without the advice of a physician, either directly or indirectly. The intent of the author is only to offer information of a general nature to help you in your quest for emotional and spiritual well-being. In the event you use any of the information in this book for yourself, which is your constitutional right, the author and the publisher assume no responsibility for your actions.

Any people depicted in stock imagery provided by Getty Images are models, and such images are being used for illustrative purposes only. Certain stock imagery © Getty Images.

Print information available on the last page.

ISBN: 978-1-9822-7176-3 (sc)
ISBN: 978-1-9822-7178-7 (hc)
ISBN: 978-1-9822-7177-0 (e)

Library of Congress Control Number: 2021914400

Balboa Press rev. date: 11/11/2021

This is for you, Daddy.
— Stevie Nicks

CONTENTS

Introduction ix

Chapter 1   Chiropractic Theory 1
Chapter 2   Emotional Pain 24
Chapter 3   Testing the Subconscious Body 53
Chapter 4   Acupuncture and Becoming a Healer 74
Chapter 5   Quantum Healing 106
Chapter 6   Yoga Philosophy 132
Chapter 7   Intention and Mental Dialogue 173

Epilogue 207
Acknowledgments 209
Endnotes 211
Index 217

INTRODUCTION

This guide is a collaborative effort to blend the two lives that I was forced to live, the two sets of eyes that I was destined to see through as a clinician: science versus intuition; trusting versus witnessing; comfortable versus fulfilling.

To continue the theme of duality, I have two kinds of readers in mind for this message. The first is someone who has very recently been introduced to the world of alternative healing. *Chiropractors, yoga, meditating, supplements, acupuncture?* The information can be overwhelming and often intimidating. *What are the benefits of this realm of care, and why does it apply to my life?* Although the purpose of learning to naturally heal is to improve our lives, we often find it during a time of personal fear, making the motive for learning unhealthy. Adapting a healthy lifestyle solely to avoid getting sick will not bring long-term peace or progress. Trust me, I know how you feel.

When this type of healing work found me, I dove in headfirst to ensure that I would not succumb to a familial disease. With that being my motive though, I learned too quickly and then desperately tried to heal with the doom of failure looming over my head. Without the proper guidance and application process, obsessions with alternative healing will only add to anxiety or a sense of losing control. If that nagging sense of feeling lost or isolated is blinding you from receiving the benefits of new healing outlets, pause, and let's move forward together.

Much of this guide will offer clinical and scientific information, as if solely directed toward other clinicians. I share education like this for the sake of raising the bar of common knowledge as well as offering hope to those who feel discouraged by the current health-care system. There are doctors with this mindset readily available to you. To find them, you will need to know what to ask and trust that there is a higher level of care that you deserve.

The second reader I have in mind for this message is the person (practicing providers included) who is comfortable with seeking alternative care but somehow feels stuck by the rising "truths" in the field. *Trapped emotions, vibrations, energy work, the subconscious mind?* Behind closed doors, many practices are implementing these techniques but cannot make false claims or advertise beyond a scope of practice. I found that what once seemed like foreign information has become normal and daily truths for both healers and patients alike. By fearlessly asking questions and displaying your own experiences with healing, you will attract the right support.

No one likes to feel left behind or out of the loop of vital information, so wherever you are along the learning curve, I hope this book helps you move forward. The guide is intended to be read, experienced, and implemented from front to back, but I know we are all on different stages of the same journey. If you are called to a later chapter, I encourage you to listen to that intuition and piece the chapters into a correct sequence for you. Do not be afraid to stop reading and take a few weeks for self-study on a topic of interest. This allows the mind-body to absorb material at a realistic pace for your life.

The material of this book is for anyone who views the intelligence of their body as something to understand instead of fear or ignore. The gifts that I will introduce are accessible to anyone because we all have an instinctual desire to improve.

Unfortunately, as a medical provider, I feel compelled to state from the beginning what this book is not for. My purpose for sharing experiences and organizing helpful information is not to convert the world to see like I do. My alternative care expertise is not aimed at undermining Western medicine but to introduce the necessity for both languages. My specific chiropractic dialect is much different from the rest of my field. I cannot speak for them all, so I offer personal experiences that have developed my flavor of practice. I cannot make definitive statements about medical or spiritual advances, but I can share the successful strategies that formed throughout thousands of successful patient visits. I feel confident in saying that this guide and its stories will speak to you. It is guaranteed to make you think and to help you recognize previously masked words or experiences in your daily life that have always been there. Even if I am not the right translator for you, trust that by being exposed to the material inside, you will have opened new doors toward finding a suitable speaker for your path.

"Healing Hands"

The human hand is the greatest tool that will ever exist.
A wealth of knowledge and history built
into cells that cannot be replaced.
A feeling of freedom, unlocking the doors of potential creation.
A recognition of patterns and invisible surface information.
A symbol of collaboration, introduction,
and synchronized rhythms.
A touch that is warm, patient, and seems to be listening.
A strength that can conquer isolation, desperation, and fear.
An invitation to trust and relinquish suffering.
An applause magnifier.
A page turner.

The spine is the hub of our life and the
link between the lower mundane worlds
and the higher realms of the self.
— Richard Rosen

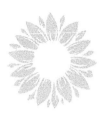

CHAPTER 1

Chiropractic Theory

My Chiropractic Beginnings

I have been asked to explain my chiropractic story many times. On the spot, my response is a quick elevator pitch formulated around my college soccer career or an interest in sports injuries following a brutal hip surgery. Thanks to the gift of writing and having the time to answer honestly, I admit that I never had that ah-ha moment calling me to a career in chiropractic. If anything, I had a string of oh-no moments from college advisers and bursar office employees discouraging my interest in the field. I was studying to be an athletic trainer when the words of a harsh professor stunted my progress. He told me that I would never get hired as an athletic trainer because I was "too good-looking" to be allowed in the locker rooms of high-level athletics. I've never enjoyed wasting valuable life on an outlet that doesn't serve me, so I quickly approached my female adviser to start scheduling a suitable path toward chiropractic medicine. She was not the mentor I was looking for, "Oh, honey, no. You don't want to be a DC (doctor of chiropractic); you want to be a DO (doctor of osteopathy)."

As a result of these discouragements, I eventually changed majors to tailor my last two years of school toward a graduate program in health care. In my new major of health and exercise science, I found beautiful and inspiring people waiting for me. Most importantly, I had a fresh adviser whose late husband had been a chiropractor (what synchronicity). Because of my background in sports medicine, she encouraged me to consider chiropractic and apply for the undergraduate scholarship in his name that would aid students looking to pursue the field. I won both the scholarship and a lifetime of gratitude for that woman. Her push was a catalyst for resistances in my life to begin melting away.

I was fighting to find summer internships in physical therapy or dietary programs until I investigated chiropractic options. I was the only student in my graduating class who requested to finish my curriculum under the eye of a sports chiropractor. I had my eye on learning from the successful doctor in my hometown of southern New Jersey. He was the man who had diagnosed my father with multiple sclerosis ten years prior. After years of unanswered symptoms and hurtful experimental medicine, this chiropractic neurologist recognized the slowly manifesting disease and referred him for positive testing. That interaction changed my family's life forever and left me with a deep respect for the field. It seemed only fitting then that I would learn under him until it was time to start my own doctorate program.

Healing Insight—Chiropractic Theory

Chiropractors spend years in postgraduate school to study the importance of the spine and its lead role in all that we do, because without it, no movement would be possible. Chiropractors are known for treating the joints of the spine, but the field has evolved into a wide array of services besides spinal adjusting, such as soft tissue therapy, rehabilitative exercises, and nutritional counseling. If you're new to chiropractic, let me fill you in on how we find the areas of the spine that need to be adjusted. A portion of chiropractors utilize x-ray radiography for a visual assessment of spinal curves, anatomy, and levels of injury or degeneration. Without film, other doctors depend on a visual assessment of motion reinforced by the information provided from hands-on joint testing known as palpation.

Every office will be slightly different in the examination process, but we are all trained to compare the quality of movement between each bone to decide if it needs more motion or should be stabilized using other techniques. Near each bone end, a joint is created in between to provide space for stable movement. Every joint in the body is lined with receptors, which are a meeting point between the nerves and the structures that they control (muscles, organs, etc.) The receptors enable the brain to perceive where in space our body parts are, what activity they are doing, if pain is registered, and what materials are needed to be successful. When motion is lost inside a joint, the brain can no longer send or receive information from that joint due to receptor interference. Over time, this disconnect with parts of your own body leads to muscle breakdown, poor balance, and injuries. But by restoring motion and balance with an adjustment, the nervous system can reach the function it was designed for; while the movement receptors work properly, the pain receptors at each joint are diminished.

> The job of the spine is to keep the
> brain alert. The moment the spine
> collapses, the brain collapses.
> — B.K.S. Iyengar

During a chiropractic assessment of joint play (motion scan), if joint motion is needed, a quick and strategic thrust is induced into the direction of motion that was lost. If the doctor's hands find excessive motion at a joint space, the stabilizing soft tissue around that region needs to be rehabilitated, and no adjustment should be provided. A hypermobile segment in the spine is a joint between two vertebrae that no longer has the correct surroundings to stabilize its motion. Damaged ligaments, a degenerative disc, improper pressure, or inactive muscles can all contribute to hypermobility. Chiropractic, combined with muscle-testing exams discussed in chapter 3, is one approach to improve the neurological activation surrounding vertebral segments. My version of rehabilitating and stabilizing the nervous system may sound extremely different from any chiropractic experience you have previously had. Within this guide, I will address deeper ways to influence what chiropractic school calls "the master system" beyond postural exercises or dietary advice. While those components are part of the puzzle, larger concepts such as mental and emotional limitations to stabilizing the nervous system should be addressed.

To ensure everyone is on the same page with anatomy, the axial portion of the skeletal system is made up of the skull, spinal column, ribs, and sternum. The word *axial* comes from *axis*, which in the body's case is a central line of reference that our anatomy rotates and revolves around. The axial skeleton is the structural home of the power cord of your body, the central nervous system. Lightning-fast electricity travels up and down the spinal cord to carry out the bidding of the brain. Because the spinal cord is safely situated inside the tunnel created by the bones of the spinal column, the success of

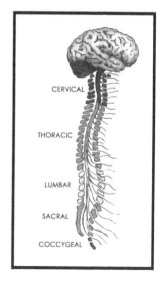

neurological transmission depends on safe movement of the spine.[1] Deviations in joint mobility can alter or influence the information that the brain tries to send to a distant part of the body via these nerve endings at each segment. It surprises patients who are new to chiropractic to find that modern practitioners can treat so much more than spinal issues, but even innovators still respect and identify the spine as the intelligent body's provenance.

While there are many specializations and niches of chiropractic care, most of the issues that chiropractors treat today are related to spinal restrictions, even if the symptoms are seemingly unrelated and distant from the spine. In a recent study published by the *Journal of Manual and Manipulation Therapy*, it was found that more than 40 percent of patients with pain in their extremities improved from spinal intervention, even if they thought there was no connection to their pain.[2] For this group of patients, their spine was the primary source of dysfunction. For cases that don't resolve after an adjustment, I funnel them into the category of a secondary or compensatory issue, meaning the spine is not the real cause of discomfort, so continuously adjusting the compensatory segment temporarily dulls the growing and overlooked issue. If the spine is truly the primary problem, most people only need the occasional manipulation for tune-ups. Going to a chiropractor regularly just to feel normal (not great) shows that the body is lacking regulation and cannot prevent a relapse in symptoms.

Throughout this guide, I will describe in detail how to improve the dialect between the brain and body. Intentional alternative care will enable you to influence nerve impulses, emotionally induced chemicals, and memory-based perceptions of your current state of discomfort or discontent. Even without chiropractic influence, you can heal many of the issues within the body. I begin with the fundamental groundwork of chiropractic's outlook on the human body because I believe that this realm of medicine is an invaluable foundation to self-healing and that every human utilizing the health-care system should be aware of its offerings. Each chapter will then introduce you to numerous techniques to complement the chiropractic lifestyle and outlook on healing.

I'm Going to Kansas City

Deep in the heart of America, I thrived in the four years of chiropractic school. My program was challenging, but it truly was a rewarding home for competitive, athletic personalities with the gift of charisma. As a younger chiropractic student, I closely identified with the athletic and masculine side of care, where success was determined by strength, speed, and the ability to regurgitate knowledge. I played soccer at the collegiate level, which strengthened my ability to perform under high amounts of stress in school. Training to earn a spot on the field felt a lot like working to obtain a doctorate degree. This athletic history allowed me to attract like-minded students as we complemented each other's growing understanding of the body in motion. I could easily relate to students who found chiropractic school following movement-induced injuries or serious surgeries. I understood how important activity was to them and how their identity had once been challenged by the loss of being able to compete. With athletes, I did not have to oversell or embellish the importance of chiropractic. We genuinely believed in the benefits because we were examples of successful interventions. Despite surgeries, fractured bones, and years of overtraining, sports chiropractic allowed these inspired students to heal when most medical programs had failed them. So, we dedicated years to learn how we had healed and how we could offer those same gifts to our future patients. We sought to understand, not mask, the symptoms that patients presented on the table.

These hardworking friends and mentors all fell within my small bubble of functional (or "sporty") chiropractic. Their bright minds helped soothe the segregation that I witnessed among current chiropractic students who were developing different styles of practice. Toward the end of the DC curriculum, students make decisions to funnel into specific classes, extracurricular clubs, and seminars based on the direction they want to pursue in the field. The temptation of successful business drives most of these selections and often skews the once creative student mindset. As professional values and business motives develop, a permanent tear severs many of the four-year friendships that once stemmed from a collective learning goal. Depending on what techniques students are drawn to clinically, divisions in philosophy and practice management are made, cementing the existence of conflicting mindsets within the field of chiropractic.

I noticed this discord early on in school and hope not to perpetuate it to younger generations of new chiropractors. I am continuously surprised to find that most people who I introduce chiropractic to are not aware of the internal variety and identity struggle within the field. Imagine if all medical doctors had to fit under the same roof during continuing education regardless of the specialty they declared. The cardiologists would love the mandatory podiatry lectures! While those limitations continue to exist, tension is bound to erupt between the passionate doctors within chiropractic medicine.

Along my path, I chose a medical and orthopedic-based route that trains doctors to treat patients for longer visits, evaluate athletic movement, and integrate care with the skills of other medical professions. I was heavily involved with the Motion Palpation Institute, who devotes their seminars to teaching integrative and strong rehabilitative interventions for chiropractors. I'm very thankful to have been a part of this organization and had access to amazing mentors while I transformed into the type of doctor that I was destined to be. Not all chiropractors agree on our role in the health-care triage, which is one of the reasons I felt called to finish this guide. I have high hopes of speaking to the minimalist in each doctor to remind them, regardless of their chosen niche, that we all have common goals and can coexist. I want to encourage the use of innovative healing techniques that, once paired with sincere human connection, will create new standards of best care.

Rowan's Imprint

Unfortunately, not everyone who seeks chiropractic care considers themselves an athlete, so as a sports focused student I was forced to find common interests with patients who preferred music, art, or religion over movement. I trusted that my skill set could benefit anyone that I made time to connect with, but I was most nervous while working with a pregnant population. I felt like they could sense the inexperienced fraud in my recommendations. I had no exposure to pregnant women or children at that time in life, so I preferred when my classmates who were mothers would cater to these patients. My perspective began to change as a student once I graduated into clinical residency. A classmate's wife and fearless mother of three wanted me to be her student intern throughout her fourth pregnancy. It was her confidence not only in our art but in my ability to care for her during one of the most important stages of life that invited the feminine healer within to safely come out of hiding.

I adjusted her with pregnancy modifications that students could only read about or witness in demonstrations, but book smarts can only take you so far. I felt her strong and intelligent body decide where "they" would let me intervene. When the joints resisted, I listened to the unspoken message of, "I'm smarter than you and don't want my naturally placed systems to be altered." She laughed at my timid touch and told me, "Bring the heat!" Beth's demonstration of faith and a female's natural ability to create life quickly removed my previous assumption that pregnant women are frail or vulnerable. What a gift it was to tangibly feel the stages of motherhood in my hands before having my own personal pregnancy. It was a true honor to take that magical relationship through nine months of care. Under the touch of healing hands, I felt not one but two numinous life forms trusting my young advice. As you could imagine, I fell in love with little Rowan on sight and could not believe the spiritual effect of holding a baby that I helped influence come into the world. If a doctor can imprint on their patients, Beth and her stunning blond son were my first.

There has been a long line of influential mothers who have found their way into my life since then, each one gifting me with invaluable clinical experiences and examples of feminine inspiration. In March 2018, over a year into his beautiful little life, our Rowan tragically passed away. To say that I was devastated is an understatement, and similarly to everyone who has been touched by this dear family, I have never fully recovered. I still struggle with the confusion of how a life that I held in my hands can no longer exist physically. Each pregnancy that I care for will always be in tribute to Beth and Rowan. Every time a recovering mother brings their new baby into my office, I hold the tiny new life and smile in his memory. He was my first. If I could go back and offer comfort to that season of grief, I would tell myself that at that exact time period, a new light had been conceived and was nine months away from changing my life permanently.

Liz and Teddy filled the void in my heart that I did not realize was present. I treated this fierce friend throughout her entire pregnancy, laughing and crying through all the ups or downs. Holding Teddy during that first week of his life while caring for his perfection of a mother gave me a strong glimpse into my own future. I felt a previously sleeping region in my body become alert and instantly longing, I knew I wanted to find my own family. Deciding to have a family threatened the clinical image of success I developed while in school. Giving myself to the people who depend on me at home would likely take away from being able to offer so much to patients and it scared me. Thanks to Liz & Teddy, I knew that that loving sacrifice was worth more than any success story at a chiropractic lecture. These pure relationships encouraged me to focus more of my clinical practice on helping other women through such a transformative time in life. Chiropractic truly gives me an insightful outlet to participate in the triumphant seasons of others' lives, and although I gravitate effortlessly toward treating athletic injuries, stories of the moms and children I have helped will hover in my memory above all the rest.

It Takes a Village

Why do children need to be adjusted? The physiotherapists from Prague who taught me about pediatric development thought it was preposterous that chiropractors manipulated kids. Until I started treating children, I thought the same thing. Children have flexible soft tissue and growth plates at the end of each long bone that are not yet fused, making the joints pliable and slightly unstable. If the traditional perception of a chiropractic intervention were true, we would be "cracking" babies like adults, trying to "pop" their stuck bony segments. Educated and informed parents of chiropractic babies get to witness the gentle impulses that a trained clinician offers to a young skeletal system. Soothing the nervous system can be done with light touch, transitory pressure, and a few recommendations for avoiding harmful parenting postures. With this intervention, crying stops, neck range of motion is restored, digestive regulation ignites, breastfeeding resumes, and the ability to develop healthy movement patterns are accessed.[3] I now love helping infants optimize their crawling, latching abilities, and rolling patterns.

Physiotherapists and chiropractors are both experts on the developing nervous system, but we speak different languages. Chiropractors have their eye on the spine and view this as the priority region of the body that dictates all motion. The physiotherapists from the Prague School of Rehabilitation are brilliant at observing the movement patterns of patients and then, by using reflexology or exercises to stimulate afferent neural pathways, re-educate the brain.[4] Afferent neurons (attacking) are sensory neurons placed throughout the body that send impulses of information to the central nervous system with what the body is experiencing. Chiropractors can use the same techniques but excel in stimulating the efferent neural pathway, the (escaping) impulses that the brain sends out the central nervous system toward the body, sparking motor movement. Both neural pathways are vitally important for a successfully coordinating body, but being the biased chiropractor that I am, driving home down a one-way, dead-end road is a waste of time. Get adjusted; heal the two-way street and open the construction barriers, receiving full access from home for a convenient and more permanent commute.

Athletic Benefits

Babies do not stay tiny for long, and there is now an influx of talented children and teenage athletes looking for new strategies to gain a competitive edge. I believe that chiropractic care is an important role for their success and prevents structural issues that would lead to discomfort later in life. Chiropractic care works well with athletic individuals because of the body awareness and visualization skills that they acquire through activity. These skills help athletes respond to manual intervention faster than someone who has no experience with trained movement.

The types of injuries that confront a sports chiropractor are inflicted during movement, so the only reasonable way to heal them is while moving. Because muscular and ligamentous injuries heal better when movement is incorporated into the recovery period, chiropractic therapies are designed to mimic your sport and the mechanism of injury.[5] Ultimately, movement should be used for more than just an assessment; it is also the treatment!

Younger patients want to develop safely as they play sports, while older patients want to maintain their activities as long as possible. Chiropractors offer athletes a diverse and conservative approach that will ensure a more rewarding participation at any stage in life. Although chiropractic adjustments cannot remove the years of microtraumas that an active lifestyle creates, they can slow the degenerative effects of training and intense competition. Restored function of the spine allows the foundational structures to withstand and safely distribute the stress created by athletic participation. For example, a properly functioning sacrum (tailbone) is an amazing shock absorber, which tries to diminish forces at the pelvis before they reach the spine.[6] When a joint is moving properly, the involved muscles and tendons can withstand the stresses they were built to accommodate. So how do you get this balanced spine and keep it?

It's called tensegrity. Tensegrity is an architectural term that describes a system in which each miniscule structure stabilizes the whole of the system by balancing the counteracting forces of compression and tension. In the body, those structures consist of elastic muscles, keystone-shaped bones, dynamic joints, and taut ligaments or tendons.[5] When the body is out of alignment and loses its tensegrity, unbalanced forces pull on the soft tissue and send uneven stresses to the spine. Without joint restoration, the prevalence of soft tissue injuries can cause bone deformity due to the shearing of muscular imbalances. With spinal and joint corrections, the body's tensegrity can function to assign safe force distribution.

Tensegrity explains why a runner landing on the heel does not fracture the bone, because tension is transmitted throughout the entire skeletal structure instead of the contact point. Warren Hammer claims, "It also explains why only paying attention to the skeletal anatomy limits a practitioner's ability to provide a dynamic solution for patients." Viewing the body as a deeply interconnected maze of chemical, neurological, and mechanical systems allows both the health-care provider and the patient to have access to optimal healing. It reminds the provider to take their blinders off while staring at knee pain to assess the big picture; Make sure to ask, "What other regions of the body are not functioning correctly that now are depending on the knee to take the extra load?"

My patients love to use the word "compensating" to describe this uneven weight sharing. I commend their awareness but continue to push the limits of their visual imagination past viewing the body as a seesaw of unbalanced weight disparities. Our rapidly adapting body is amazing at finding new efficient patterns to make up for a lifetime of abusive postures and emotional interactions. Compensation is one step into the world of understanding tensegrity. A system that achieves tensegrity is yet another step closer to true relief, or peace, which is the goal for my care.

Breaking the Ice

The science and techniques above are so important to understand as a young doctor. What truly matters though, is being able to communicate clearly and help patients realize its importance. Let me be the first to explain how messy, experimental, and challenging it is to develop that voice. The first year after a doctorate program in school is an overwhelming collection of firsts for new clinicians. It's possibly the first time they'll move far from home, are no longer a legal student who's handed loans to live off of, the first time they have to sell a skill set to others for money, and the first time they'll worry about their personality as much as their clinical experience (which is minimal fresh out of school). This year is a confusing jigsaw puzzle of a time when young doctors test the waters to decide how to present ourselves and which of the many techniques that we learned are the most effective for each visit.

I accepted my first clinical position after graduation in a sports practice near the heart of Tulsa, Oklahoma. I spent three years in the athletic style of chiropractic practice, during which I was exposed to less traditional alternative care such as emotionally induced pain and yoga therapy. During that time, I devoted social media efforts and my online presence to sharing the message of chiropractic's potential and why it deserved a seat at the big table. Overwhelmed by the lack of common knowledge in a field that I had dedicated so much time and money toward, my message softened, and I aimed my efforts at things I could control: slowly educating the person on my table, watching one light bulb turn on at a time. I used each new patient to hone my communication skills and create a flexible approach to introduce foreign concepts in an easy, accessible way. I regurgitated my in-depth reading, shared fun success stories, and utilized the knowledge of authors much smarter than I to cement a point. Throughout this process of learning how to kindly approach the subject of alternative care, I have found that reaffirming words, reinforced by the safe actions of healing hands, will always attract those who need it.

Along the way towards healing, you may meet people who have answers for your questions and who have questions that you can answer.
— Julia Pelvin,
The Healing Magic of Forest Bathing

Tulsa Time

The discussion of chiropractic science comes up in nearly every interaction I have with new acquaintances. It is my lifestyle, my language, and my currency. I love to subtly ask everyone about their chiropractic experience, and although I typically expect negative responses, I rejoice in the success stories that have found their way to me. In response to my probing, I've heard it all: "My chiropractor said I have one short leg"; "I was told I have the worst neck she's ever seen"; "My neck is actually a reversed curve and will never get better." If prompted, I use gentle words to rewrite some of the damage that a hurtful provider (in any field) has ingrained into the deep subconscious mind of a suffering patient. *Subconscious*—the things you do or think without realizing it.

One response that I struggle to forget was from an athletic rock climber who moved from St. Louis, where she left a beloved family chiropractor. Once in Tulsa, she found a new doctor (highly rated on Google) who, while examining her pelvic alignment and spinal curve, reported that her pelvis was so misaligned that she wouldn't be able to have kids until it was properly corrected with chiropractic care. My mouth dropped open, and my eyes bulged as she relayed the story. I briefly composed myself and remembered that each patient interprets our dialect differently. I hoped, for the sake of my profession and the other patients who utilize that specific doctor, that he did not say such a blunt and life-altering statement without any medical tests to support it. This strong and healthy woman had no prior accidents, illnesses, or cause to question fertility while in his office. His scare tactics were the exact reason she never returned to him as a patient—or any chiropractor since. I assured her not to give up on our proud science and to keep trying to find someone who matched her goals and communication style.

Proud Like Sarah

In the world of health care, I ask that all providers take the weight of their words very seriously. In chiropractic, we do not normally interact with patients suffering from life-threatening issues, but that shouldn't make our communication style any less accountable. In a moment of fear, we (the patient) revert to early seeds of medical advice garnered from our parents or a childhood doctor. Even as a trained musculoskeletal doctor, when I feel any soreness in my right hip, I still hear the warnings of an old hip surgeon as he casually told me, "You'll need a hip replacement when you're older." The image that that man implanted in my head at nineteen lives on despite my athletic capability and professional understanding of joint injuries. Without testing and without second or third opinions, I do not believe in making blind definitive statements that could influence someone for the rest of their life. I am incredibly careful with the words I use to relay a diagnosis and suggested care plan, yet as a young doctor, it is challenging to find your big-girl voice without making too many mistakes along the way.

One of my favorite chiropractic success stories started off with this type of tension. Sarah was a young girl who had woken up with a numb right arm three months prior to meeting me. She could not lift it, use her fingers, or contract any muscles without aid. She was genuinely concerned, as were we all, that this was a permanent issue headed toward an invasive, exploratory surgery. At her first visit, her dad put me on the spot and asked if I could fix his daughter. He was a straight shooter, and I wanted to answer him with candor. I have never been a fan of the word *fix* in medicine.

With healing, and life in general, avoid the allure of being fixed. While answering Sarah's dad, I made sure to avoid offering false hope until we went through a care plan and established progress. What I could assure them of was my willingness to tackle any structural or functional issue within my skill set as well as knowing when their time and money would be better spent at a different style of medical provider. I would keep them informed each step of the way as I discovered what was happening. That honest answer was enough for them to trust my judgment while staying compliant during a three-month experimental trial of chiropractic, rehabilitation, and spinal decompression. Their diligence and the collaborative effort of the many styles of care set Sarah free of her phantom arm numbness.

On one of her final visits, she walked in my office, chest held high, and showed off her restored ability to put up her own hair into a ponytail. Neither of us will likely take such a simple display of independence for granted again. Her story is a favorite of mine not only because we cleared her back to cheerleading and avoided the exploratory brachial plexus surgery but because it was an interaction that I was extremely proud of. I handled and directed the communication carefully and represented the best of what chiropractic can offer—no fluff, just results and healing hands.

The Healing Touch

It is such an honor to be in a medical field that still touches people. Many modern physicians have conformed to an insurance-influenced bedside manner that keeps them at a safe distance from patients and limits all interaction to short, financially beneficial appointment times. As a chiropractic acupuncturist, I have a different approach on how to observe the body. I am enormously proud of the autonomy of my career and how it offers each provider the opportunity to meet eyes with a stranger, listen to their goals, and then collaboratively explore the issue with consistent contact.

As a new clinician, I was surprised to witness how many people use chiropractors to fulfill their need for human touch—a primitive desire. I caught on, reminded the patient how naturally resilient and capable they are, but obliged them by spending most of my treatment's attention on touching their tense, muscular tissue. Functional chiropractic attracts a variety of dirty work, but someone must do it! In one visit, my gloved hand could be stripping the inside of a patient's jaw muscles as I mentally heal from the sight of the previous patient's abdominal surgery scars, not knowing that the person in the lobby waiting for me is going to show me a horrific foot that survived an ultramarathon that previous weekend. Tears, vomit, sweat, curse words, and laughter have all come out of patients as they witness the depths of hidden symptoms that rise to the surface in response to human touch. A chiropractor who uses their hands as the priority intervention can feel how much trust exists between the two of you. As you relax into the healing hands that calm a back spasm, realign your pregnant pelvis, or offer a condolence, I relax alongside you. Without words, the right set of empathetic and skilled hands should remind you, *you are safe to heal here.*

Finding the One

Lisa Rankin, author of *Mind over Medicine*, encourages providers to collaborate with their patients from the first meeting; "Somewhere in the intersection of hope, optimism, nurturing care, and a full partnership with the empowered patient, a recipe for healing lies." When it comes to finding the right chiropractor, I have a few recommendations. Look through local websites until you find an attractive fit, and then call ahead and ask these five questions:

1. How long will I be in contact with the actual doctor?

    • Ideally greater than ten minutes each visit. Fifteen to twenty is even better. This style is often more expensive, but you will heal faster (fewer visits in total), develop a deep relationship with the provider, and have the time to learn about the true nature of your body's imbalances.

2. Does the doctor adjust with their hands?

    • A doctor who manually adjusts uses the best tools for information, their healing hands. They should have other forms of adjusting for lighter or smaller patients, which may include tool-assisted adjusting, but you want someone who knows what to do with their hands first and foremost.

3. Are there memberships or prepaid treatment plans?

- I prefer a doctor who helps you quickly and efficiently and attempts to do so permanently. Scheduling follow-ups should be based on progress, not an upfront package. The presence of memberships also correlates with a style of doctor who won't spend much time with you each visit.

4. Does the doctor release patients?

- Releasing patients is the goal for a functional-minded chiropractor. We want to diagnose you, educate you, and then the ultimate goal—release you. An office that does not release patients is a specific business model that correlates with quick appointments and lots of return visits. Life happens, so monthly maintenance is necessary, and a new care plan may start if you suffer another injury. Then again, the goal of that new cycle is to diagnose, treat, educate, and say goodbye!

5. Does the doctor offer any services for soft tissue issues?

- Our bodies get misaligned while moving muscles, ligaments, bones, and the pressure chambers in between them. To heal permanently and efficiently, both the soft tissue and joints need to be treated. Sports chiropractors are best at offering soft tissue release, rehabilitation, and reeducation to complement chiropractic adjustments.

The golden rule for finding the right provider is to keep trying! Do some research, try another office with a different style, and have faith that the guidance you need to heal yourself is attainable. Don't hesitate to move on from a current doctor if you are not receiving the results you deserve. Due to the intimate nature of the field, I find that people become fiercely loyal to their chiropractor. Maybe they see a family friend or "a really nice guy." Even without permanent results, these loyal patients will avoid the inconvenience of changing to a different chiropractor. I trust that you will know when you have found the right fit for you. The provider's words, listening eyes, and knowledgeable suggestions will all complement the safe hands that hold your body on a day where pain builds up beyond your threshold of tolerance.

Review Questions

1. What is your current impression of chiropractic treatment?

2. Does that stem from a personal experience or something relayed to you by friends, family, or social media?

3. Do you feel obligated to continue seeing the same chiropractor out of friendship or routine? Wouldn't it be nicer to find someone who thinks similarly and can heal your issues so you don't have to continue going so often?

4. Have you asked your chiropractor what seemingly unrelated conditions they are capable of treating?

5. Make a list of barriers that your chiropractor should honor to make you feel safe:

    *
    *

6. Write down your current perception of pain and what limitations seem normal and permanent?

    a. Example: "I have incontinence because I've had kids. It's normal."
    b. Example: "I have a bad knee from surgery. I'll feel it every day for as long as I live. It's permanent."

7. Build the perfect provider in your mind and invite them into your existence.

    a. Include location, price, specialty, experience, personality, bedside manner and so on.

8. What is a daily creation that your hands form?

9. What is an important interaction that your hands have enabled?

10. Whose is your favorite hand to hold, and what emotions does that touch evoke?

It does the world no good for me to be seen as
someone whose ideas are "outside the box."
My mission is to make the box bigger so that these
concepts are part of our culture and way of living.
— David Perlmutter MD

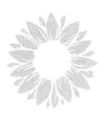

CHAPTER 2

Emotional Pain

I have spent many years dedicating my life to learning so I could offer clinical support to others, preventing both life-limiting injuries and mentalities. Physical support is the gateway to earning someone's trust and is why I introduce it first in this guidebook. Like many other areas of life, my chiropractic practice has changed and evolved many times. With unique mentors and heavily focused yoga training, my clinical style has morphed into a dynamic system of emotional healing, intuitive corrections, isometric muscle rewiring, and subconscious reeducation. I utilize my favorite portions of manual techniques like adjusting, soft tissue release, and rehabilitative exercises, but there can no longer be one way to treat the masses. Each person I see will have a different experience in the office. Each treatment is unique and is altered to match the personal expression of every *body*.

A Reminder from the Dead

Coming from a chiropractic setting, I could only accept tangible truths about the body. Because my love language is physical touch, I excelled in hands-on classes that dealt with one-on-one patient care. In comparison, I worked hard to absorb enough chemistry, radiology, toxicology, physics, and neurology to earn high marks. All the material we learned in anatomical courses of study were then reinforced in dissection labs where numerous cadavers would offer each student a personal experience with the structural components inside the body. Cadaver lab teaches you what pictures and drawings look like on the inside, what systems are physically connected to what, how strong bones and fascia are, and how cruelly human beings can treat their own bodies.

One of the most eye-opening experiences I had in the cadaver lab came to me the day a deceased woman was assigned to my group, forcing each of us to witness how temporary life truly is. She was thin, tanned, and could have been a mother to any of the young students around the table. Even after the classic medical student precautions of covering the face and groin before dissection (the two creepiest and most lifelike areas to witness on a dead body), I was deeply disturbed by the woman in front of us. I hadn't been squeamish in the lab any years prior to this class, but I was starting to wake up and notice subtle things that my classmates easily looked past. As they started to rush through the day's assignment in hopes of getting to the gym faster, I stared at the neon pink nail polish left on her cold but kind hands.

I mentally cursed the company that prepared the body and questioned how quickly they could have removed the nail polish. Such a simple act could have made this interaction easier for me and allowed me to pretend I was cutting through a fake mannequin. Although it would have made that week easier for me, in the long run, I'm glad they left her perfectly painted nails alone. To see such a tiny yet substantial sign of previous life opened the door in my mind to question which style of doctor I planned to be. I don't see much difference between analyzing a cadaver and how many practitioners currently view their living patients—a big body of static bones, muscles, and tissue lying on the table waiting for their intervention without participating in the process. I wish

I knew the young woman's name or what intervention could have prevented her heart disease, but I'm grateful for the constant reminder while treating patients each day; signs of deeper life are always visible if we care enough to look for them.

Healing Insight—Emotional Pain

The modern patient now has amazing access to an abundance of online information, giving them an empowering chance to enter a doctor's office with knowledge of their condition and the potential mechanism that caused it. This abundance of information can be a blessing and a curse if not guided to safe sources by a personal physician who understands your specific diagnosis. My teachers jokingly warned us in school that our biggest competition in practice would be "Dr. Google" and "Dr. Pinterest." Like many other modern alternative care providers, I love that my patients come in with a general understanding of their body and what went wrong during daily movement. This baseline of self-awareness and knowledge allows me to skip fundamental conversations and focus our time on things they would not have learned without a physical experience guided by healing hands.

An informed patient heals quicker, which is why I'm not afraid to push the limits of what a patient can comprehend is happening within their body. Using physical demonstrations to reinforce foreign concepts, together we raise the standard of what is considered "normal information" about the human body. The most common conversation that sparks confusion in my office is how surface pain can be emotionally driven, and not solely from harmful movement. Most patients who walk into my office struggle to accept how tangible and intangible parts of the human body can both create physical pain. They've never been exposed to deeper signs of life in their own body. Throughout treatment, I guide each patient through a series of discussions and interventions that introduce what many healers coin emotional pain.

I divide the care of emotional pain into three traditional categories: inflammatory chemical pain, psychosomatic pain, and metaphysical pain. Depending on which audience I am speaking to, I explain the stages of emotional pain differently. The dialect should match the goals of the population and offer support to the mindset of people who are in attendance. In other words, read the room. During lectures and workshops, I ask that mixed groups stay ambiguous and try learning alongside the different professions. Most neurologists do not subscribe to yogic philosophies, just like a room full of chiropractic students would shun me if I started a lecture describing how to influence the spine by communicating instead of manually intervening. In a yoga setting, I discuss emotional pain as energetic disruptions of prana. To psychologists, I refer instead to the unconscious mind and studies about motivated reasoning. In my office, I use the word *psychosomatic* to describe pain that originates from the brain, not from an injury to the body. I spend most of my clinical time treating inflammatory-triggered injuries that stem from a chemical trigger, such as stress or a harmful diet. While performing anti-inflammatory modalities and mechanical interventions, I explain the concept of chemical pain.

Stage One: Inflammatory and Chemical Pain

I first introduce patients (and anyone who initiates a health conversation with me) to the idea that surface pain has a deeply rooted cause by using the discussion of chemical inflammation. Not many people will argue the connection between a swollen injury and imminent pain. Swelling is a localized sign of inflammation, which tells us that the systemic first responders in the body are fighting to regain equilibrium or homeostasis. In a homeostatic body, chemical hormones, inflammatory markers, nutrients, and antibodies are ideally regulated and functioning correctly. When an acute (fresh) injury occurs, the levels of systemic markers change drastically to resolve the issue and may demonstrate surface-level signs of distress, such as high temperatures, swelling, bruising, or throbbing.

A situation that is harder to recognize on the surface is caused by the symptoms of chronic (long-term) injuries or inflammation. Repetitive cycles of chronic pain disrupt the body's ability to find peace and regulate itself. Endless cycles of self-healing and continued damage leaves a toll on the body in the form of vascular plaquing, tendonitis (chronic inflammation of tendons), skeletal tissue scarring, and joint degeneration. In a chiropractic setting, I believe this is vital information for patients to understand how their aching pain could stem from molecular inflammatory wars. It surprises them to learn that things beside movement and body positions can trigger repetitive spinal dysfunctions or physical pain. Lifestyle factors such as anxiety, emotional imbalances, dietary choices, and hydration levels can alter the chemical health of the muscles and ligaments that support your spine. Chiropractic care complements all these areas of health, which is why I am so honored to have it as my foundation of medical training. Instead of healing a specific ailment, chiropractic works to increase a general sense of well-being to bolster immunity and help patients thrive. Still, chiropractic is only one tool on the toolbelt of many ways to heal our human experience.

Chemical pain is a category that clinicians use to classify a patient's injury as something that has stemmed from a chemical imbalance in the bloodstream, such as unregulated hormones, diet-induced inflammatory chemicals, parasites, and pathogens. Dr. David Seaman describes in his work *The Deflame Diet* that chronic chemical inflammation from these systemic markers can lead to the development of chronic pain, diabetes, depression, heart disease, and cancer.[1] In my office, I view a molecular imbalance as a two-way street in terms of pain generation; it can either be the cause of structural discomfort or the result of misaligned structural functions. To determine if pain or chemical influx came first, doctors use a series of diagnostic questions and tests to spot red flags that would help us lean toward one of the categories. During manual therapy, the body is aligned to restore the proper balance and function of musculoskeletal structures. Those corrections aim to calm local areas of inflammation that reduce the need for chemical stress and subsequently resolve most surface pain. When a thorough conservative care plan does not resolve or alter the pain, we must assume there is another component at play—the chemicals surrounding the involved tissue.

Megan's Health Scare

I once struggled to help a woman in her forties who had fractured her midfoot while working in her garden. Megan hobbled into my office with a boot prescribed by her orthopedic, which she had already been wearing for six to eight weeks. I offered her rehabilitative services to improve pain and strengthen the surrounding joints while she followed the non-weight-bearing recommendations of her orthopedic. My goal for this extremity injury was the same for all functional injuries: balance the pelvis and spine, reduce asymmetries in muscular patterns, decrease improper stresses that disturb the injury site, and accelerate the healing process. Like many patients in my style of practice, the woman had already emailed me a long explanation of her injury so I would be caught up on her story. I skimmed the email beforehand to respect the exhausting medical process I was sure she'd already gone through but knew I'd have to ask her my own questions to piece together a version of the story that matched my expertise.

Each provider looks for different components of your health history. I wanted to understand more than how she got hurt and if she suffered a previously similar experience. I needed to understand why this injury was mentally scaring her and which emotions were exacerbating her symptoms. Without addressing those components, the physical side of my interventions would continue to hit roadblocks and have a confusing response to care.

Upon questioning, the woman said, "I have four weeks to get out of this boot so I can go skiing with my family on a trip that we've been planning for years." *No pressure,* I thought in my head. As she continued, she told me about going to her doctor months ago, complaining of idiopathic foot pain (an unknown cause). They dismissed it because she was not an active person and disliked exercise; there was no cause to suspect a movement injury. She eventually stepped on a stick in her garden, which caused her foot to make a large "snap." The film done at that time produced a fracture in her fifth toe, mandating a non-weight-bearing boot. She denied any history of osteopenia, but I started working on her stress fracture with a skeptical eye about the density of her bones and altered the strength of my spinal adjustments.

Over the care plan of a few weeks, we were able to improve her functional ability and pain, yet in her follow-up imaging with the orthopedic, her fracture had not healed at all. She was devastated and had to accept her inability to freely enjoy her upcoming trip. After detailed imaging, we came face-to-face with the true roadblock to healing—severe and systemic osteoporosis. No other doctor had taken the time to review her imaging findings, so the emotional aftermath was crashing down on my plate. Through tears and apologies about her anger, she looked to me to explain why her efforts didn't amount to our expectations. I empathetically reminded her of the goals we were targeting but it was disappointing to see her go through this. I can't heal bone density, but I did help her recognize how this current failure would become a long-term blessing; without her injury, she may have continued living under the assumption that there were no chemical imbalances within her body, allowing the distress to escalate toward more threatening injuries. Her pain and emotional irritability were the first signs from her body that deep systems were failing and needed help.

Another grouping clinicians use to categorize an injury is called mechanical pain, an issue in which the joints, bones, or fascia/muscles are the primary issue. When a patient truly has a mechanical issue, they should respond quickly to chiropractic manipulation, massage, or other manual therapies. When there is an underlying systemic issue, such as imbalances in the blood/hormones/organs, normal surface treatment won't satisfy the deep source of inflammation for long. We don't always feel signs of chronic inflammation until the dysfunction rises to the surface as a musculoskeletal pain or systemic disturbance. Like my skier, by the time we complete a trial of care on a seemingly mechanical surface issue, it is too late to catch accelerating systemic inflammation.

To complement the manual services, I recommend that all patients seek a health-care provider such as a Doctor of Osteopathic Medicine (DO), a chiropractic internist (DABCI), a naturopathic doctor (ND), a registered dietician (RD), or someone who works with functional medicine. These specialized providers will address your internal imbalances, refer if necessary, and utilize natural sources to safely establish an anti-inflammatory chemical environment. Anyone living in a pro-inflammatory stage (very inflamed) will not heal as well or as fast, regardless of the manual intervention they seek. Routine internal tests and care plans with these providers will prevent a lot of the injuries that wind up in my office!

Stage Two: Psychosomatic or Phantom Pain

After patients witness their own progress with physical pain in response to cleaning up a diet, removing a pathogen, or restoring hormones, they gain a new perspective on the body's ability to talk to us. I tell them that pain is simply a conversation between the subconscious body and the person trying to translate it. The subconscious body is the portion of our automatic brain that controls systems without our knowledge and remembers all the things we do not have time to focus on. For example, we don't tell our heart to pump or the lungs to breathe, yet that control from the subconscious brain is in a constant state of activity and communication. During lectures and patient care, I use the subconscious body to introduce the concept of psychosomatic pain, a term used to describe how mental processes can result as a physical symptom even when a physical ailment or condition is not structurally or cellularly present.

There may always be a component of chemical irritation and physical malalignment, but a patient categorized with psychosomatic pain (mind influencing the *soma* or body) has a condition mostly aggravated by a mentality or emotional distress. This term is becoming recognized within the orthopedic medical community and is helping to set new standards of what is considered normal care. The manual therapists who take the time to recognize that mentality and emotions play a large role in the physical health of their patients are already a step ahead of their colleagues who continue to view the body as a machine (easily manipulated by forceful manipulation, surgery, or drugs). By embracing this concept and spending a brief portion of each visit on emotional health, patients will witness the control that they have over mentally produced pain. In return, this saves money for the health-care system and offers peace of mind to people who end up in the emergency room with back spasms after a stressful fight with their boss.

The subjective (self-reported) experience of pain is built from both the state of our body and the context of feelings that surround those sensations. The brain catalogs movement by closely intertwining motor patterns together with the memory of how the movement feels. I call it an emotional pattern. In a pain-free range of motion, the brain remembers simplicity and ease, so the movement memory is stored as a positive experience that, when evoked, produces helpful and happy chemical reactions. Past the point of a pain-free range, your body sends updates to the brain to prepare itself for a position that it has previously associated with difficulty or discomfort. If the body has not correctly healed an injury or benefited from the necessary care, those preparations trigger inappropriate muscle firing or chemical stimulators. The mind will then use resources based on fearful memories to avoid another injury. So how do we alter that?

Throughout schooling and continuing education, I have been taught the definition of the term *psychosomatic* without an advised way to heal it. It seems that addressing its existence is professionally acceptable but approaching a way to treat the phantom pain is hearsay or reckless. Witnessing a sign of distress and then avoiding its implications qualifies as negligence in my eyes. Not all providers are in the right headspace or scope of practice to help heal stress-induced pain, but luckily, medical offices are not the only outlets that can heal those imbalances. I believe life has a way of healing us naturally, thanks to supportive interaction with loved ones, transitional stages of growth, and our daily ability to choose healthy lifestyle habits.

Physical therapist and medical author Annie O'Connor says that personal contact and emotional support play a big role in coping with life stressors, which influences how we all experience levels of physical pain.[2] The fear of injury, reinjury, or being in discomfort prevents us from moving past old injuries, even if the conscious mind forgets the impact it had on us. The systems in your body that directly communicate with the brain exist to respond to changes in your arousal. Feedback loops and brilliantly detailed regulation cycles respond to our ever-changing moods and chemical instigators. On demand, as the body anticipates movement, the necessary systems signal arousal hormones (like adrenaline or cortisol), metabolism processes break down nutrients for fuel, and neurological excitement prepares to execute the motion.

Physical anticipatory reactions to arousal are professionally researched and easily accepted, but how can we justify the mentally triggered reactions that occur even when movement does not? Like an athlete who mentally visualizes their event before moving, the brain is practicing efficient ways to combine emotional and physical experiences of motion. My kind of athlete, an intuitive and aware mover, does not practice visualizing movements alone but also anticipates how they are going to feel mentally during different parts of the competition. Using this creative visualization process and empowering affirmations, they create an endurance for the fear, doubt, and unanticipated pain they will encounter. I believe we all do this, regardless of our athletic involvement. During dreams, daydreaming, and creative journaling, we offer our bodies a chance to assign emotions and feelings to the minutiae of the day. Becoming aware of the stressors that take a toll on our physical experience is the first step toward realizing we can then alleviate the reaction with positive responses. When we recall memories of safety, comfortable temperatures, good communal meals, and carefree activity, enjoyable sensations rise from the depths of the body via neurochemical chain reactions to our conscious surface. In contrast, during seasons of adversity, we often wonder where those euphoric memories are hiding and how to dig through layers of suffering to reach them.

The Limbic System

Numerous regions in the brain contribute to pain suffering, including the anterior cingulate gyrus, the hippocampus, and the

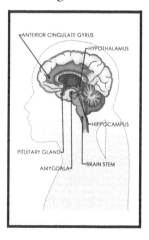

amygdala of the limbic system.3 The brain's limbic system is a sophisticated region that manages emotions, memories, and subconscious stimulation throughout our day. The hippocampus is one portion of the limbic system that is responsible for creating new memories and perceptions of experiences. When negative memories or anxiety drive our daily routine, the overproduction of cortisol and glucocorticoids weaken the

34

synapses of the brain to inhibit formation of new ones.3 Synapses are the communication sites between all nerves and allow our bodies to rapidly transfer information. Without the ability to form new nerve synapses and neurons, the hippocampus in the brain cannot form new healthy, happy memories. It is stuck dwelling on existing and possibly depressing memories, so this cycle of negativity is hard to break.

The amygdala is another portion of the limbic system that augments emotions and fearful stimuli in response to memories. Repetitive triggering of a stress response oversensitizes the amygdala and wears down the hippocampus.[3] Bad experiences get programmed in the amygdala without a clear record of what happened triggering ongoing anxiety even after the threatening circumstance is over. The unconscious mind is anxious and agitated, while the conscious and surface mind has no clue why. Portions of the limbic system are situated inside the prefrontal cortex of the brain, sometimes called "the seat of our consciousness." This cortex pieces together our thoughts and actions to match mental goals. It's interesting then to speculate how guided conversations and visual healing can remind our patients of positive and achievable health goals. By understanding the role of this system, we can utilize it during meditation to bring our conscious mind closer to the depths of the unconscious body.

The limbic system of the brain works closely with the influence of psychosomatic pain because it is one area involved in emotional memory production, specifically reflexive emotions. Regarding movement, the amygdala of the limbic system stores the emotional component of a memory as it gets cataloged. Until a movement that contradicts or improves the original experience comes along, the existing belief remains like the filed memory and produces an anticipated response.[4] For example, until someone in my office experiences what a pain-free forward bends feel like, they will continue to believe that when they bend forward, it will reproduce the symptoms that they have come to expect during such a movement. I call the process of contradicting or improving a memory experience "rewriting." For movement, rewriting a pain experience, no matter how long someone has suffered from pain, is liberating. The first time a patient bends forward without debilitating back spasms, they realize their body is capable of healing and that pain is temporary. It requires more conversation and persistent strengthening to convince the mind that the previous pain will not return.

> When we have fear or anxiety the brain sends negative signals and we are overpowered by such feelings. If we have faith or confidence in our body, the brain sends positive signals to promote healthy movement or healing. In medicine, we call this the placebo effect but in ancient yoga it's called sraddha.
> — Kausthub Desikachar

The nervous system depends on the structural support and successful ability of the musculoskeletal system (any tissue in the body that supports motion). Maintaining a healthy structural system enhances the ability of the nervous system to perform, monitor, and induce healing. Yoga came into my life after suffering from another debilitating soccer injury. I couldn't walk let alone run so I needed to heal both my discouraged mind and body. The practice of yoga is one of the most in-depth ways to improve the nervous system, which is why, as a chiropractic student, I was so drawn to its benefits. I wanted to learn by witnessing the changes in my own body before asking my future patients to trust such a dedicated process. The deeply intricate patterns of breath and muscle movements in a yoga sequence takes the body beyond daily ranges of motion and normal postures. These gentle extremes of range can excavate the memories of emotional pain that has been built into the building blocks of our tissue near that once limited joint. Like a tree that grows in an outward spreading layer of rings, humans lying on a chiropractic table may seem physically healthy and strong on the surface. But if the tree is cut into layers horizontally, we can witness the seasons of nutrient detriment or damage in the rings from a year that the overall health of the tree resisted and grew past.

Where Emotions Live

Our cells are constantly regenerating to remove unhealthy seasons of life, but the history of the emotional and physical stress experienced at the time can remain in the building blocks of our physical tissue. In between the signaling tissue of the nervous system, a microscope will magnify a chemical interaction that is important to understand for my interpretation of emotional pain. Neurotransmitters are biological chemicals that are sent to ignite a reaction within the gaps of nerve endings, known as a synapse. The current theory by neurobiologists is that memories live at a synapse. This cellular theory suggests that lasting memories are dependent on a healthy network of neural connections and will fade if the synapses degrade.[5] The late Dr. Candance Pert, author of *The Molecules of Emotions,* believed that biochemicals such as neuropeptides are the substrates of emotion and therefore exist to interpret the sensations of the entire body. They are not the thought, but they move with it to serve as a portal of transformation. She reminds us that "we can no longer view the emotional brain to be confined to the classical locations of the amygdala, hippocampus, and hypothalamus. We have discovered other locations with high concentrations of almost every neuropeptide receptor that exists, such as the dorsal horn, or backside of the spinal cord."

Chiropractic adjustments intimately influence the dorsal horn of the spinal cord. The delivery helps to fine-tune synapses at each nerve cell which prevents them from fading. This is one way that chiropractic care also prolongs the joint degeneration caused by traumatic interventions or normal aging. Healthy joint movement and consistent activity keeps the body's regulating systems fresh. Researchers at the University of California, Los Angeles proved in their 2015 study that the brain remembers how many baseline synapses should be at each nerve cell and will work to restore that number if they are destroyed.[6] The findings strongly suggest that neuronal synapses are a crucial component of memory but that ultimately, a memory lies in the neuron itself. Our brain alone holds 86 billion neurons! That is a lot of emotional, sensational, and movement-driven memories.

What the body holds onto is not yet clear and reproducible in research. If you ask any practicing clinical doctor who uses their hands, such as movement therapists, massage therapists, or yoga instructors, they'll all have a story about witnessing a spontaneous outburst of emotions in a previously neutral patient following a manual intervention. A chiropractic adjustment can restore a deep spinal restriction that may have been present for many years, and the instantaneous rewiring of the nervous system's communication at that spinal segment is shocking. By releasing the lost memory of all the synapses that provide information to the brain, it's like breaking a dam and flooding the brain with lost memories, giving it a sudden ability to speak to that segment's spinal nerves, their motor units, and every organ system that the segment innervates. Dr. Candance Pert believed, long before society was prepared to agree with her, that "virtually all illness, if not psychosomatic in foundation, have a definite psychosomatic component."

Stage Three: Metaphysical Pain

> When we knot our muscles, clench our teeth,
> or tie our guts in knots, it does little for us
> but cause pain, raise blood pressure, and
> create more noise in the nervous system.
> — Michelle Levy, author of *Mindfulness,*
> *Meditation and Mind Fitness*

Most of my patients and colleagues can understand the neurology and physiology of psychosomatic pain without any need to further question the vague term. To a learning doctor, the term suggests that no physical ailment is present in the tangible body and that the true issue is a mental one. Few clinicians feel that a pain mentality or "emotional reality" lies within their skill set, so they transfer the responsibility away to another doctor, starting the doctor-patient relationship from scratch. Throughout school, my hands were trained to become a chiropractic clinician, but I viewed each lecture through the eyes and ears of a yoga student. Under that philosophy, healing that goes beyond the physical and into the mental realm is called *metaphysical,* a word that would never leave the tongue of a medical professor. When I began practice and increased the number of daily interactions I had with people, I started to witness healing that I could not classify as mechanically or chemically induced pain. I now needed a term that would explain the confusing cases where patients would attribute pain relief to faith, emotional breakthroughs, and shared energy from a "healer." I came to coin this category of pain as metaphysical; an imbalance of the body that stemmed from a mechanism that was not tangible or molecularly identifiable to the common clinician. It is hidden from the physical body that we see.

While developing a system to identify a metaphysical case and successfully care for it, I used observation skills and intuition to identify patterns in the patients who had already benefited from intuitive techniques. Most of them were nervous at a deeply neurological level and even during gentle treatments demonstrated signs of sympathetic distress, such as twitching eyes, crossed legs, and breath retention. They were usually the kind of patient who looked uncomfortable lying on the table and laughed in embarrassment each time I touched their guarded body. To address what was harming these patients, it would require a flexible and intimate style of care that I had not developed yet.

I struggled for months and embarrassed myself in front of early patients who felt I was losing sight of the initial reason they came to see me. Not everyone wants to share their emotions in an unfamiliar setting, and it's even more rare that a busy provider will make enough effort to cultivate such vulnerability. In those early stages, I allowed my youth and inexperience to limit my ability to help people who were struggling with life events I had not experienced yet. I felt confident working with young women and loved helping children, but that was only a small portion of my practice population. To contribute to the emotional healing of the masses, I remembered the goals of my foundational training and decided to only tackle the metaphysical cases that I could speak to, such as the physical sensations left over after near drownings, life-threatening surgeries, or car accidents.

Each success story built my confidence and reaffirmed a decision to abandon my previous frame of mind. The small failures or inability to help a few people didn't hinder my journey to find more answers. Investments in courses, yoga certifications, and hundreds of books were time and money well spent because I had a "lab" to fine-tune the newly acquired material. In my mind, education without application will soon be lost. Learn, apply, and put your own twist on the information until it matches your beliefs, becoming a permanent part of your knowledge. The more I believed in the power of our ability to influence the subconscious mind-body, the more my patients believed in me. As trust grew, results started happening faster. My ability to recognize and then release emotional pain grew exponentially once I had enough tangible proof to stop clinging to my need to understand it. I was not making claims outside of my scope of practice, tricking people for money, or exposing them to danger. I was simply asking them to pay attention to which emotions triggered pain episodes and what would ideally alleviate that stress hiding in the body.

I dove in, shedding a lifetime of fear of how others respected or viewed me. I handed tissues to hundreds of people as I scurried around the table stretching and probing their tissue. They healed. I healed. We healed together. More people found the office for a chance at deeper healing. They returned the next day with their kids and spread the word to friends. Everyone wanted a taste of these experiments. What was shocking pain relief on their side of the table was equally as shocking to my hands and inexperienced body.

Metaphoric Pain

> You can't see yourself because
> you're looking at your judgements.
> — Louise Hay

Throughout my education of emotional pain and learning to treat the deep nervous system, I was introduced to the existence of what I began to call metaphoric pain. Bundled into the metaphysical pain category, metaphoric pain is a collaboration of physical symptoms that result from a figure of speech. We acknowledge that the subconscious mind speaks to us using imagery and metaphors during dreams but are less familiar with its continued messaging system throughout our daily thoughts. The body, influenced by our cultural saying and values, becomes an object that can represent or symbolize a figure of speech, such as "I've been stabbed in the back by my uncle" or "I have the weight of the world on my shoulders."

The people who suffer from unresolved traumas in life can hold these metaphors in their subconscious mind until the surface of their body represents the imagery, tangible sensations included. I was unable to grasp the existence of metaphoric pain until having patients of my own who benefitted from exposing the metaphor that they were living with. I have found that when taking a jump outside the normal realm of medical care, you must experience the results in your own treatment room, under your own hands, before genuinely believing it can exist. The idea that a simple conversation, mental imagery, and a verbal affirmation could remove pain that a patient has reported to have for many years cracked the medical foundation that I stood upon. In those unsettling moments, I had to decide what my true purpose was as a doctor; was it to preach the guidance of textbooks or research articles or to offer patients in pain a glimpse into their own ability to relieve suffering? The quantitative markers of functional progress and improved strength that I documented after these healing sessions dissolved my quest to understand everything about the body. I left the office each day questioning, "What else are we capable of?"

Head over Heels

The symptoms of metaphoric pain will present differently for every person, and it is up to the provider to creatively translate the picturesque, emotional injury that the patient describes. The first case of metaphoric pain that I was brave enough to address was with a woman who, while describing her back pain, was using words that brought my attention to her posture. In a medical setting, we would call her lumbar curve a "sway back," meaning her pelvis was shifted further beyond the line above her ankles, making her low back excessively arch and her torso sway backward from her center of gravity to compensate. While I recognized the posture, I couldn't ignore the circumstances she mindlessly mentioned were causing her fear of moving forward in life. Looking at a patient using the symbology of a metaphor changes the eye of the observing doctor. Instead of plumb lines and uneven spinal stresses, I saw Jean's gut leading her life direction while her head and heart retreated from the decisions. I asked Jean if she had any upcoming challenges with transition. She said that she had recently removed an important person from her life based on her gut instincts and intuition. I asked her why she normally resorts to instinct over logic, and she responded that she didn't trust her own mind. "It is too conflicted with the advice from other people." With the risk of sounding crazy, I asked her to recognize her standing posture and to resist me from pushing her forward. As I lightly pushed her midback with one finger, Jean almost fell forward!

This young, healthy woman should have much better balance than what she displayed, and we both laughed at how weak she felt. With a few prompt questions, she decided what emotional behaviors she needed to witness in the man she released from her life. Once doing so, she felt she'd be able to trust him enough to make decisions that were heart based, the compromising connection between instinct and logic. I let her have some personal time to think and witness other areas in life that she was disconnecting her emotions from while I silently mobilized her ankles. Only minutes after the first test, I pushed her midback forward again, only to be resisted by a fully stable spine. Jean turned to me with wide eyes and said, "Oh my God!" Her lumbar curve had reduced closer to what I would consider normal, and the tension in her midback had resolved. Alongside my normal manual intervention, these are the deep conversations that I wholeheartedly believe should be considered best care. Treating a patient's body without addressing the mind's influence is temporary and superficial. If we have the means and the heart to face the true seeds of imbalance, why shy away?

Over the course of three years, I eventually found the confidence to combine metaphoric pain with physical pain on a regular basis. I allow my diagnostic brain to dance with the creative mind while I work through a patient's muscles and joints to identify patterns that build a metaphor. There are endless examples of these metaphors, but the patterns I see most or are most memorable include:

- Feeling betrayed or "stabbed in the back" that results in a sharp stabbing pain in the ribs
- Wanting to have conviction and "grow a spine" resulting in slouched, unstable posture
- "Dragging my feet" resulting in achy, heavy legs
- Idiopathic chest pain referring to the back after "my heartbreak"
- Stiffness in the back when forced into a situation of "my back is up against a wall"
- Bilateral wrist pain that did not respond to conventional care from "my hands are tied"
- Trigger Finger from refusing to "pull the trigger" on a decision in life.

Releasing Shame in Tory's Body

Not all the metaphors are light or sarcastic. Some of the most challenging appointments I have held space for included revealing a metaphor to a patient that crossed the line into deeply personal traumas. Using my best professional judgment, I would demonstrate how the metaphor was affecting their physical body at an appropriate time, make some improvements, and then refer them to a therapist to further address the mental barriers. After a patient's consent, there were a few times that I invited a willing therapist into the treatment room to witness our treatment. They would talk afterward about potentially working together if the patient thought they were a good match. Bringing a therapist into an environment that is already comfortable for a patient has been a successful strategy to encourage hesitant women to seek counseling. One of these young women had severe tailbone pain, which usually indicates a weakness in the stability of the pelvic floor. Her midline muscles were nonexistent; both inner thighs could not contract, her unilateral core muscles could not resist me, and any other muscle test that would pull away from midline was graded a 2 out of 5 in strength. Because I had a good relationship with this patient and knew she wasn't suffering from any surgical interventions, I felt it was appropriate to rule out that she hadn't experienced any abuse or sexual trauma beyond having her first child three years ago.

The metaphor that came to mind was "keep your legs shut." The patient said she had never been mistreated sexually but came from a deeply religious family that shamed her sexuality. Even as a young wife and mother, the mentality that sex was wrong affected her marriage and physical response to opening her legs. With cautious wording, we discussed the beautiful sensations of bringing her innocent child into the world. I watched her body relax as that familiar example of pure love sunk in, banishing any doubts that the pelvis, the part of her body that created something so pure, could be anything but good.

Immediately following our healing conversation (that took all of five minutes of my treatment time), her muscle testing became a 5 out of 5 in strength, producing only minor pain in her tailbone. We continued with manual care to aid the irritated ligaments and spinal misalignment, but that quick restoration of proud strength gave her relief that has now lasted for two years. This would be the first of many women in the Bible Belt who would confide in me about their disconnect with this sacred part of their body. I became an active referral base for pelvic floor therapists and sex therapists in town so that together we could resolve the physical and mental limitations these women experience each day.

There are many authors and healers who have dedicated their lives to sharing the potential healing capabilities of metaphoric pain. Due to my professional obligation, I cannot make medical claims of guaranteed patterns or condone trying to heal life-threatening conditions using mental affirmations alone. I admire the ease and conviction of some of the world's most popular innovators in this realm, such as Louise Hay, author of *You Can Heal Your Life* and *Heal Your Body*. To learn more about the many patterns of metaphysical pain, I encourage you to research her message. Other intuitive authors, such as Bradley Nelson or Joe Dispenza, are chiropractors who have stepped away from the clinic table to spread a message beyond their reach. In doing so, they are not able to practice anymore due to conflicting scopes of practice and insurance-based limitations of what chiropractors can do. This limitation happens in every medical field; chiropractors are not the only doctors realizing that emotions are speaking to them during care.

To decide if what you are experiencing can be considered emotional pain, I encourage you to seek a health-care provider who will ask how your emotions affect your current conditions and then offer resources to relieve them. Recognizing and deciphering which metaphor is harming the body is part one of the challenge; the second part is then releasing the mental prison that keeps us chained to the metaphor. Like all holistic aspects of the body, there are physical and mental components to this category of pain. I rely on the skills I was trained to utilize during manual care and have learned to complement them with developing intuitive skills for the deeper aspects of pain. For some, physical intervention is all that is needed to encourage a body away from metaphoric or emotional pain. I find that these cases are normally patients who have not previously trusted someone to touch or help them. For those who regularly receive manual intervention like massage, chiropractic, or acupuncture, they have cleared most of the superficial work that can be released by physical stimulation and need emotional guidance to resolve deeply seeded imbalances.

Kristin's Emotional Release

Kristin is a strong and caring woman who found her way into my office in the early stages of my clinical development. She had dealt with lower back pain for ten years that was exacerbated by her career as a nurse practitioner. In our first visit together, as we spoke about her previous surgeries and feminine health patterns, we found a correlation between her increased back pain and her monthly cycle. At this point in my training, I did not have the confidence or skill set to heal anything beyond her structural discomfort. When Kristin told me that she had suffered from invasive surgeries to correct irregular periods and cycles of painful endometriosis, I made sure to ask if she had those conditions monitored by her ob-gyn. To most chiropractors, documenting that conversation and recommending some helpful supplements covers what can and should be done for Kristin's symptoms. Knowing that all structural pain can benefit from an improvement in joint stability and neurological rewiring, I refused to transfer the responsibility of this caring woman to another provider without even trying to intervene.

In Kristin's case, the junction where her thoracic spine and lumbar spine met was extremely restricted. This heavy epicenter of nerve roots, once regularly firing, controls so much of the lower abdominal organ systems and pelvic floor muscles. I adjusted this segmental restriction in Kristin with a heavy "thud." After the "crack" of the spinal cavitation, Kristin's face gasped for air while her legs shot up into the air and her stunned body let out a wave of tension. I backed away and observed the quickly changing response and worried that my inexperienced hands had harmed her. As her body started to accept the correction a few moments later, she melted into the table with a peaceful look as if prepared to take a long nap. I asked, "How's it going? Calming down?" She did not answer me, but through closed eyes, I watched tears pouring down the side of her temples, puddling near a piercing on her cheekbone. The intense neurological release subsided. The adjustment was exaggerated by what we would both describe as a release of deeply restricting and trapped emotions. She sat up on the table and, despite the surface-level sensation of my lingering adjustment, had zero signs of back pain.

I continued to treat Kristin for years following that incident, and we both laughed about the change in perspective that it taught us. She still swears by that one adjustment and how its deeper intention cured her chronic low back pain. As a more experienced practitioner, I now prefer to identify and resolve painful memories prior to a manual intervention. Making peace with a previously traumatic sensation sends calming neurochemical messages from the brain to the entire body, activating the parasympathetic nervous system and its control over physical systems. Having the time to create space for these conversations is a permanent component of my treatment now. The connection created from vulnerable and caring conversation creates an outlet to fully receive healing benefits, reduces discomfort during the intervention, and improves the time frame of which the correction holds its effect.

There are many ways to decrease stress in life, like mindful movements, meditation, and pain relief. My treatment as a manual therapist is devoted to bringing the nervous system back to ease so that patients will benefit from those recommended activities. Calm lights, approachable body language, and encouraging words all contribute to removing emotional pain. Follow the next steps to address emotional pain at home and talk to your health-care provider about any lingering symptoms that concern you.

Healing Emotional Pain without Physical Stimulation

Step 1: Express your current stress and how you believe it manifests in the body. Identify the home of emotional discomfort in the physical body. Common areas include stomach distress, head pressure, hip clenching, or shoulder tension.

Step 2: Characterize the emotional discomfort to help the brain process the sensations. For example: "It's a deep and cramping tightness in my chest. On the right more than the left currently, but it moves around while I am sitting in meetings."

Step 3: Acknowledge that pain is a message from your deep consciousness.

Step 4: Identify and resolve the trapped emotion. This may come from a quick gut instinct or a flash of some symbology in your mind. Trust whatever words pop up. There are many ways to spark an emotional release, and it is important to do it while in a safe environment where the shedding can be supported and properly resolved. Therapists, yoga practices, breathing exercises, support groups, and self-help books such as *The Emotion Code* can assist you.

Step 5: Replace trapped emotional pain with positive sensations and experiences. In comparison to how the body feels in step 2, visualize and invite the opposite sensation to occur in your body. For example: "When I stand on the beach, I feel my chest loosen as my shoulders open so that my breath normalizes to match the breeze."

Review Questions

1. Assess the physical pain you have been experiencing recently.

   a. Was it the result of a movement or posture?
   b. How does the pain respond to certain foods or medicine?
   c. To gain more of a connection, what health behaviors can you try to alter this week that your pain may benefit from?

2. Take mental inventory of the emotional state of your body.

   a. Scan the body for tension. It can potentially hide in the jaw, the gluteal muscles, or the intestines. Follow it if it moves. Where does the sensation land?
   b. When you breathe, are there areas that resist expansion or hurt to try?
   c. Does the breath hide in the top of your chest, or can it find safety in the bottom of your abdomen and pelvic floor?

3. Visualize how your body looks during a time of stress.

   a. What body language, age, size, and activity does that represent?
   b. Do you recognize yourself?
   c. What body language can you instead visualize that represents a true, healthy you?

4. Work through the steps on the previous page for one specific area of discomfort in the body.

5. Make a plan to connect with a provider or new self-help book that will address chemical imbalances and accessible ways to bring them back to equilibrium.

The unconscious mind of the body seems
all-knowing and all-powerful.
In some therapies,
it can be harnessed for healing
or change without
the conscious mind ever figuring
out what happened.
— Candace B. Pert, PhD

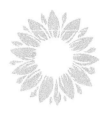

CHAPTER 3

Testing the Subconscious Body

Throughout my healing journey, I have witnessed a surge of unlicensed bodyworkers rise to the surface of mainstream health care. Although they are not recognized by insurance companies, bodyworkers are the first level of healing access for many people who avoid the medical system. Luckily, chiropractic is a normal intervention for someone with this mindset, so my diverse patient population introduced me to many of the techniques I'll discuss in this guide. As I focused on improving my chiropractic skills one patient at a time, the missing techniques that I'd need to make a true difference in their healing found me! Through conversation, the person on my table raved about a healer that came into their life and how wonderful it would be for me to meet them. I was amazed to hear how much money my patients would pay out of pocket for alternative areas like private yoga sessions, intuitive readings, or energy work. They believed in it fully. It seemed as if they went to a medical doctor for their blood, the naturopath for their hormones, the chiropractor for aches and pains, the therapist for relationships, the massage parlor to be touched for an hour, and then the holistic bodyworkers to have their soul cleared.

So, I made a few appointments; I wanted to experience emotional releases from deep fascial work, the meditative calm from a float tank, shaking out the bad vibes from sound bath healing, having my eyes read by the iridologist, and my deep subconscious memories tapped into by a "muscle tester." I fell in love with the physical sensations that came from such intimate bodywork, and I felt called to learn more about the diagnostic tools that these gifted healers used to pull the true me to the surface.

Healing Insight—Muscle Testing

Manual muscle testing is taught in many manual therapy professions such as sports medicine degrees, chiropractic, and physical therapy. This style of diagnostic tests gives the doctor objective information on what muscles of the body are weak and/ or cause pain when being utilized. Sports medicine doctors or athletic trainers refer to this method as a "break test technique." It describes the process of applying an overloading pressure against a stationary muscle as the patient is asked to contract or resist. The provider then stabilizes the local joint and tries to "break" the strong hold of the patient's position. Muscle weakness and pain during a test like this can indicate a soft tissue strain or joint instability. Muscle weakness in the absence of pain can also indicate nerve damage.[1]

Like I discussed in the first healing insight, a chiropractic adjustment's goal is to restore motion through a joint restriction in hopes of improving the brain's coordination of that joint and all its parts (nerve, muscles, receptors, etc.). A manual muscle test shows the clinician where the brain has lost its control over a muscle system or synchronized movement pattern. With the proper joint restoration, the brain should effortlessly be able to fire muscles at that level of nerve control for full strength and endurance. I use these tests throughout a patient visit to demonstrate an immediate effect of our adjustment's intervention, which a patient will notice as a strong change in neuromuscular control and restoration of pain-free movement.

When the doctor uses testing like this to assess the body, they are solely addressing structural information such as muscular control and joint stability. The diagnostic movements won't evaluate energetic or emotional information that could be contributing to the patient's condition.

The muscle testing used by many types of alternative providers will look like orthopedic training, but the large difference is the intention behind what they are looking for. Instead of functional quality or pain, an energy healer believes the body will prevent strong muscular control if the energetic channels that run through that muscle are storing trapped emotions or pain memories or have been decided by the ego that they are less than normal. A healer's muscle testing will look less like the widespread analysis of muscle testing and more like a repetitive attack on one muscle, called an indicator muscle. An indicator muscle becomes a baseline of strength to answer the provider's questions in a yes or no fashion.[2] A yes results as crisp, full-strength muscular contraction, while a no is indicated by a weak or stuttered firing pattern. The variables that influence the results of indicator muscle testing make it impossible to recreate between practitioners, providing low reliability for research studies. What are the benefits? Why do so many practitioners trust the results of testing? Let's explore the practice methods and terminology of both manual and indicator muscle testing within alternative care providers.

Learning to Understand the Subconscious Body

The term *subconscious body* gets casually tossed around in a lot of alternative healing outlets, such as massage, yoga, and acupuncture. Without accurately describing the phrase, this deeply hidden sign of innate life is often dismissed as esoteric or taboo. When I use the term subconscious body in this guide and during patient education, I am referring to the very real autonomic nervous system, its control center, and the life force that connects the mind with the body through this coordination. The autonomic nervous system (ANS) is one of the two branches of the peripheral nervous system (all nerves outside of the brain and the spinal cord). The ANS is the portion of neurological control that we do not have voluntary control over, meaning I cannot ask my heart to stop beating or target my kidneys during an exercise like I do with my glutes. The autonomic system supplies the blood vessels, dura mater, periosteum, ligaments, and intervertebral disks, all vital structures that support the more popular anatomy of the body.[1] The ANS is a window of opportunity to explain an underlying intelligence that constantly communicates with every human experience in the body, all underneath our awareness.

To make things more confusing, the ANS is again split into two systems, the sympathetic or parasympathetic nervous system. This categorization is often explained as the *fight-or-flight* section of the nervous system, compared to the *rest and digest*. I will go into greater detail about fleeing or freezing in later chapters, but for now, understand that while we cannot control the ANS or the subconscious mind-body, we can influence it and learn to better connect with its subtle signs. This is a vital pillar in my philosophy for educating patients, and I believe it is a gift that goes far beyond healing from a current injury.

The spine can be viewed in paired pieces known as a vertebral segment. The term *vertebral segment* describes two articulating vertebrae, the fibrous disc in between, and the pair of spinal nerves that escape the spinal cord in the space between them (see image 3). When the segment is restricted in motion, due to poorly aligned surfaces, unequal pulling of the surrounding musculature, or traumatic interventions, chiropractic theory believes that the spinal nerves cannot function with ease and efficiency. There are thirty-one pairs of spinal nerves along the spine (See image three), each in charge of organizing organ systems, muscle movement, and feedback from the brain. At the base of these spinal nerves, their nerve root —the portion of a segmental nerve that is closest to the spinal cord —has two components.

The first is a somatic (voluntary) portion that controls skeletal muscles and receives sensory input from skin, fascia, muscles, and joints.[1] This is the information that athletic injury and orthopedic muscle testing seeks to understand. The second portion of the nerve root controls the organ systems and is part of the autonomic nervous system (involuntary). This is the information that indicator testing seeks to expose.

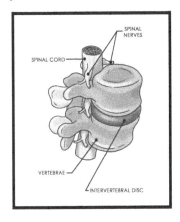

I studied the autonomic nervous system in school but had little intention of applying that textbook knowledge to each in-person treatment. I found out very quickly in clinical practice that the meticulous training for eight years of college had only skimmed the surface of the nervous system and all its potential. For many doctors outside a neurological diplomate, this complex system is viewed as an inaccessible maze that will never be under our control. In chiropractic, the nervous system has been deemed the *master system*, a strong term equipped with equally strong risk of disruption. For the young and panicking doctors, muscles and bones are easier to grasp, which is why I remind patients that I am a glorified mechanic. Even seasoned clinicians who get caught up in their normal routine and further away from neuroanatomy training in school avoid incorporating the nervous system into each daily visit. Without muscle testing, I was guessing, feeling, and cracking in hopes of resolving pain and soothing the nervous system. Muscle testing was the first doorway after graduation that offered an obtainable chance to witness the nervous system's constant presence in our human experience.

What's The Big Deal

The original muscle-testing protocol that I learned was designed to correct movement systems and identify true causes of dysfunctional movement patterns stored in the brain.[3] This technique perfectly complemented an orthopedic style of training and made sense to my neurologically trained eye. It served as both an assessment and the treatment for the athletes in my office. Repetition was key, and I quickly found my groove, testing poorly coordinating muscles alongside the chiropractic interventions that improved the imbalances. Patients loved to see the results and could often feel the strength changes immediately following a spinal adjustment. Muscle testing offers a provider a neural pathway to demonstrate the motor control changes in the cerebellum of the brain. This is the lower center near the brainstem that coordinates and stores all movement programs.[3] Using a muscle test to correct movement validates (to both the patient and provider) the strength of chiropractic care's ability to rewire the nervous system. I depended on manual muscle testing to help demonstrate how temporary the disruptions of our body can be.

I was very satisfied with the results until I realized that not all spinal corrections could restore muscle strength. If the primary issue that causes pain is truly a spinal restriction, then the adjustment should permanently help. If it doesn't, focus must be placed on the limiting adhesions found along fascial slings that control that site of pain. Fascia is the innervated fibers that bundle muscles together and is found to enable long slings of movement producing muscle groups. Freely sliding layers of muscle and their fascia allow for instantaneous firing patterns and pain relief in compensatory systems.[4]

To restore poorly moving slings of soft tissue and the bony structures that support them, many doctors utilize muscle screening techniques like SFMA (selective functional movement assessment) and FMS (functional movement screen), which are wonderful baseline tests to create a direction for a treatment plan.[5] All this anatomy and protocol information pours out of a clinician's head while we quickly identify what will best help the person on our table. In the cabaret style of modern chiropractic, the best of the best develops a seamless ability to jump between manual disciplines without missing a beat. But even with all the training at my disposal, there was pain I couldn't resolve, people I desperately wanted to help and stubborn muscles that refused to stay strong past a few days.

It was a hard pill to swallow when chiropractic—my foundational area of study—failed to be enough. I personally witnessed the limitations of a one-track mind and sought out accessory styles of care to add to my clinical toolbelt. With a hunger for obscure knowledge, I chose to work in an office environment that encouraged each doctor to view the body as a deeply intelligent temple that longed to heal. With the help of mentors who had struggled through personal journeys of their own, I was granted a fast pass to higher learning and dove headfirst into a world of subconscious healing. Muscle testing was a major component of this new direction.

One alternative healing technique that came knocking on my clinical door early in practice was applied kinesiology (AK). Developed by George J. Goodheart in 1964, I was exposed to a brief level of this style of chiropractic by a very introverted, brilliant student who has gone on to become an intuitive, all-encompassing asset to his medical community. AK doctors were the first group of chiropractors who blew my mind and made me defensive about the style of chiropractic I had chosen to pursue. As if in a deep trance, these methodical doctors dance around their patients, poking, prodding, adjusting, and muscle testing everything involved. They understood patterns of muscle activation and dysfunctional neurology at a lightning pace that revealed the holes of my education and possibly a superficial style of learning anatomy. Why I reference the technique in describing my work is that AK uses a combination of manual muscle strength testing (challenging different muscles in the body to compare neurological control and firing quality/endurance) and the energetic philosophy of acupuncture (meridians, trapped emotions, organ functioning) to evaluate the body in a much deeper way than any of my mentors had tried to. The treatment system I adapted uses pillars of this style of muscle testing to demonstrate how emotions, organ-referred disruptions in chi, and mental perceptions affect the physical body's pain, weakness, or discoordination.

Manual Muscle Testing Fine-Tuning

You've got to get the fundamentals down,
because otherwise the fancy stuff
is not going to work.
(Randy Pausch, *The Last Lecture*)

Like any other skill, practice makes perfect! A trained professional uses their extensive anatomy training and finesse to properly perform the work of muscle testing. Taking webinars or training programs for testing techniques is the most efficient way to learn both the science and application of the art. At home, intense study of the origin, insertion, and actions of muscles in the body is a vital baseline of information to successfully apply manual muscle testing. For body work and energetic muscle testing, a different category of skills should be developed to successfully implement the work in your services. Confidence and finesse are two areas that will ensure the success of muscle testing. Confidence stems from preparation; proper study and training offers an unshakable foundation to fall back on when live patient interactions make you nervous. Confidence also influences your communication style. The better you can explain the necessity of your work and how muscle testing enables it, the more compliant the client will be.

Confidence does not mean strength! The nervous system can only process so much information at once, so lessen its load by taking excess stimuli from the provider's body out of the equation. Learning to add resistance lightly and smoothly during muscle testing allows the provider to receive more feedback from the patient's body alone. Consistent timing and pressure application creates efficient motor patterns in the provider's body and leads to higher-quality results.

Position is also vitally important. Be systematic and do not rush or cut corners. Make every effort to keep variables between the final check and the original testing prior to treatment. If I use my right arm the first time to resist the muscle, then after treatment, I make sure to check my work while standing in the same place, using the same arm, and with the patient in the original position. Most skeptical minds are looking for reasons not to believe your care, so take unnecessary opportunities to validate their concerns off the table by staying systematic.

To help witness their nonconscious mind, I teach skeptics how to find signs of an instinctive intelligence within them. In my world, feeling is believing. I have been taught to believe that the autonomic nervous system controls our deepest functions, but I didn't believe we had a connection with that life force until feeling it for myself. Feeling—a sequential process of acknowledging a physical sensation, trying to translate its purpose, and then witnessing a physical alteration in response to that mental inquiry—is believing. Some people call it luck when hip pain or a stomach cramp vanishes after mentally soothing the nervous mind, but to those in the bodywork field, we believe that our internal dialect has something to correspond with. The voice of reason, our consciousness, the gut instinct—these are all terms to describe this invisible sidekick that influences our daily lives and physical direction. When the body answers back, everything about your mental and sensory experiences will change; eyes turn their focus inward, ears learn to hear sensations as clearly as audible sounds, and the fear of physical isolation melts away.

Energetic Muscle Testing

One of my favorite slides to present during lectures is a series of diagrams that show the breakdown of tissue mass into its tiniest elements. Beyond the building blocks of skin or organ tissue are individual cells specifically made for the function of that bodily system. These cells communicate with one another through various mechanisms of travel, vibrations, chemical reactions, or morphological changes, but one common interaction that maintains the continued functioning of all living cells is through electricity. Each cell can be further broken down into charged components that are maintained by an energetic field of perfectly balanced electrical pull. Every microscopic energy field combines to form larger, buzzing masses of collective fields. The body is an electrical circuit on legs. Although seemingly large in relation to subatomic particles, our individual circuit is barely on the radar when compared to the entirety of our ecosystem's energetic field. Chapter 5 will specifically address the science of vibrating cells and the rise of quantum healing, but for now, understand that each living species offers a unique electricity into the world, and as we blend to influence the environment's field, we are influenced by its alterations in return.

Placing the energetic field of another substance within the energetic field of the body can cause a temporary and measurable change. The energetic substance interfering with our personal field (another person, animal, natural food source, etc.) can complement or disrupt the field that our electric bodies thrive in. I now use muscle testing while treating to demonstrate this change but can remember how hesitant I was to subscribe to any technique that utilized an electrical theory as a student. I have never been one to blindly accept insight from a teacher without questioning why, so I started doing my own review of available research to formulate an explanation that proved the potential value of muscle testing.

When I stumbled upon the galvanic response phenomenon, I felt like I was putting small connections together between physical and energetic healing. The galvanic skin response (GSR) was one of the earliest tools used in psychological research and offers a method of measuring the electrical resistance of the skin. Electrodermal activity (EDA) is the current preferred term for electrical conductance changes of the skin in response to nervous system activity, and it demonstrates the changes in the autonomic nervous system regardless of obvious signs of change on the body's surface. The testing clarifies how the brain's responses to experienced stimuli are influenced by emotion, attention, and cognition, which affect our behavioral decisions.[6] The polygraph, also called a lie-detector test, is an apparatus that measures physiological variables such as heart rate, blood pressure, and respiration rate. Polygraphers believe that when people are asked threatening questions to which they respond by lying, physiological changes will occur that will show up on the polygraph record. In response to a stressor, GSR or EDA measures an objective indication of autonomic nervous system activity in response to observed stimulus. It is ultimately a measure of emotional arousal, where excitement from a stimulus will react with a strong galvanic skin phenomenon (a strong spike of neurology). If no memory arises and the person is unmoved by the verbal/visual stimuli, they won't display skin excitation or a change in temperature (omission of a neurological spike).

For indicator muscle testing, I encourage bright minds to consider the galvanic skin arousal as part of the discussion in explaining the brain's ability to answer yes or no on the surface. The strong spike of neurological arousal indicates an excitement toward something beneficial or desirable, guiding the provider toward a "Yes, please give me this." The lack of response in neurological activity goes below baseline strength of neutrality, demonstrating something undesirable or a "No, I don't want this."

O-Ring Muscle Testing

Like most seekers who stumble into the world of healing, muscle testing was introduced to me from the healing hands of mentors whom I considered gifted. For two years, I watched these clinicians perform amazing feats of pain relief, movement progress, and functional restoration in ways that seemed unnatural or superhuman. They taught me to channel my own expertise and intuition to define a style of muscle testing that I felt confident implementing. I found confidence from literature and resources beyond the men who taught me. I found that there are many different styles of muscle testing. The most accessible and easily recognized is called the O-ring test (see image 4). The Bi-Digital

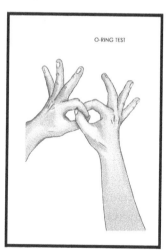

O-ring is a muscle test developed by Dr. Yoshiaki Omura, a Japanese cardiologist. His work presents a muscle test as a diagnostic procedure for alternative medicine and is based on the belief that hands hold an extremely sensitive electromagnetic field that can be measured using an electromagnetic resonance test, similar to the EDA. The form of the O-ring test that I learned first has a patient create an O with his or her fingers. The clinician evaluates the patient's pain or condition by asking questions and then trying to pry the fingers apart.[7] According to the patient's finger strength following each question, Dr. Omura believes the subconscious body will dictate the necessary direction of care.

Try for Yourself—The Ring Test

1. Make the O: To start, create an O with your index finger and thumb on both hands. Intuitively choose which hand will be the break hand and which will be the indicator hand. The break hand will initiate the force after questioning to try to break the opposite ring open. The indicator O will try to resist and stay closed for answering.

2. Acquire a baseline: With a calm mind and steady hands, maintain a grip on the fingers that is consistently firm but not aggressive enough to lead toward fatigue. To gain a baseline of muscle strength in response to something true, the first statement or question should prompt an answer without emotional attachment. Asking a name is a great question to start with because the response is something unbiased, neutrally stimulating, and re-creatable. Example: "Is my name Marina?" If the indicator ring fails while trying to resist opening, this means the nervous system took over and offered a "No." If the indicator hand successfully resists being broken after the question is asked, the result is considered a "Yes." (Note: This will be challenging to do if you have injured fingers or wrists, and the brain will not want to continuously stress the affected region.) If the muscle goes weak, that is considered a sign that the body does *not* want the stimulus. If the indicator muscle stays strong or gets stronger after the question, that would be a sign that the body wants that stimulus. Other fun baseline questions include asking a favorite food or color for a firm yes.

3. Assess the subconscious body: Once you have the sensation of what a true strong yes feels like, it's time to move on to your personal and creative system of muscle testing to resolve imbalanced joints, healthy stimulants (oils, supplements, high-vibrational book selections, etc.) or emotional influences. A detailed description of this process can be found in Bradley Nelson's book, *The Emotion Code.*

Muscle Testing Fine-Tuning

Like all the techniques that I now believe in, I learned to apply this style of muscle testing in my own life to witness the benefits firsthand. I slowly learned to read the delicate responses of a muscle test's yes or no. I fumbled, cursed my gullible mind, and questioned how much influence I had on the results. It was not until I experimented using the O-ring tests on patients that I learned to trust that the results were legitimate. Legitimacy in my mind came from reported or observed changes in pain after following the instructions of the indicator's responses. If the muscle test guided the session to restoring motion in the ankle, I altered my care in that direction instead of focusing time on the primary area of complaint, such as the shoulder. Even if I couldn't explain with certainty how the muscles were participating in the body's desire to heal, people got better. After fifteen minutes of therapy on the distant ankle, I came back to the initial painful sight to find zero issues with the shoulder. Without having quick access to the brain, I could have wasted weeks of time and the patient's money while trying to silence the compensatory region of pain.

Following the galvanic response concept, the subconscious body will only respond with neurological stimulus to answer yes or no. Stick to simple yes or no questions to not confuse yourself during care. For example, a confusing question to direct care would be "Is the foot included in this injury?" It offers a vague answer and will require many follow-up questions to narrow down a proper protocol for movement care. A better question for muscle testing would be "Is the right foot a priority to adjust today?" Notice how I altered the question to keep the focus of the answer within my skill set.

I believe that acquired knowledge sets a limitation for successful and reliable muscle testing. My training has prepared me to be an expert in musculoskeletal interventions. I would not believe the results of a muscle test if I was asking a patient's body about their liver physiology or hormone production. Collective consciousness can enhance the personal limitations of the provider because a muscle test is an electrical combination of two systems, two lifetimes of experiences and skill sets. Still, the provider needs to have enough of an understanding of the patient's knowledge to ask relevant and efficient questions. My biggest advice when learning to muscle test yourself or others is to refrain from asking objective and biased questions. For example, "Does your husband love you?" That panic-provoking question will instantaneously alter alarms in the brain and influence the response before the provider can pull on a muscle.

A muscle-testing provider that I sought for treatment reminded me that this style of work is considered "emotional reality." The answers are dictated by how my brain, my truth, personally views a situation. What is true in my mind could be a false reality for most others. It is also extremely hard to remove yourself from human interaction without inserting your own assumptions into the treatment. It takes a lot of practice to stay detached from the results of testing and an amazing amount of humility to recognize when the provider is not in a healthy headspace for clear results that day. Many novice muscle testers don't follow these rules and scare themselves when their own fingers respond yes to the prompt, "Do I have a tumor?" Millions of neurochemical components react to even hearing the word *cancer* and will immediately influence the answer due to fear and dread. I remind muscle-testing students to keep it simple and don't take advantage of questions that could lead to self-doubt or harmful mindsets. Asking an inappropriate question will limit your confidence in the ability for truthful intervention. Do not test the future or things you know you shouldn't rush the answers to. Anything that has not happened yet is pure anticipation and will offer an unreliable result.

For medical providers, never ask a question in which the response will vaguely hint toward a diagnosis. Stay within your scope of practice and remember my encouragement in chapter 1 about taking the weight of your words seriously. Use your studied tools and training to diagnose, and if needed, implement muscle testing to fine-tune the care or get past a plateau in progress. For bodyworkers, yoga teachers, or anyone learning the art of muscle testing outside a health-care outlet, please learn what a scope of practice is and refrain from dabbling in any area that might offer false hope or mental harm to a client prior to referring them to an appropriate physician. This is an accessory tool to better connect with patients and to further understand the intimate communication between the body and the mind. While learning the language of this mind body, ask simple questions, keep a pure intention, and trust that you are making a difference.

False Results and Arguments Against Muscle Testing

Indicator muscle testing is unfortunately too subjective to study effectively. Because every doctor has different strengths and personalities, it is impossible to recreate the same testing protocols and results between numerous practitioners. There are also too many moving variables in the patient to produce reliable study methods. Beyond acquiring a baseline, many students have trouble maintaining consistent results. There are many factors that can offer false positives during indicator muscle testing, so to minimize the confusing variables, the tester should place themselves in a position that offers the patient a safe and neurologically calming position:

- Avoid hovering high over someone or being in a daunting posture while testing.
- Minimize visual distractions for both the tester and the tested.
- Use kind and nonaggressive contact.
- Avoid placing the client in a similar position of recent injury or previous trauma.

Until a widely accepted protocol and description develops, the muscle-testing clinicians will have to rely on verbal feedback, personally felt progress, and improved function to determine the success of their tests. For those of you who are new to muscle testing, please let me offer the counterarguments to this technique so you have the skills to spot and avoid a provider who inappropriately uses the technique. Beyond bad form or physical application, there are many ways to poorly test muscles. There are tricks that will immediately cause muscles to go weak that an uninformed patient would not know to question. Common tricks include:

- A testing provider grabs a limb at the wrist or ankle and compresses the carpal bones, making the patient's muscle fatigue naturally.
- The cervical spine being axially compressed to increase intrathecal pressure and limiting the spacious flow of systems supporting a muscle group.
- The most common, pushing resistance on a limb in a distal direction. *Distal* means further away from midline,

while the term *proximal* means closer to midline. Pushing a limb in a proximal direction during muscle testing will create increased stability, giving it strength, something a provider would do at the end of the session to show apparent improvement. For providers learning to be honest and consistent, I stress learning systematic, orthopedic muscle testing first.

Why I Accepted the Gift of Muscle Testing

As a student learning to become a sports chiropractor, I was threatened by indicator muscle testing and was convinced that the practitioners using the tool had to compensate for a poorly trained ability to heal someone in an orthopedic way. If I hadn't learned muscle testing from one of the brightest sports chiropractors in the country, I never would have committed to learning how to implement the technique. This initial disdain came from my first experience with a muscle-testing doctor while I was a student in school. He was a successful chiropractor and a known salesman for a nutritional supplement company. I felt taken advantage of and was too shy to refuse paying for the large number of supplements that muscle testing "said I needed." I have learned to better understand the implications of successful nutritional support in techniques such as applied kinesiology but still err toward this recommendation: find a skilled practitioner who uses muscle testing to create physical results that are indisputable and not in the doctor's best interest. Indicator muscle testing should not be used as part of an elaborate scheme to abuse the sales of a product or service.

Despite living in a society where we all have separate interests and motives, one undeniable commonality that every human can agree on is a tangible, positive sensation experienced by the physical body. We are unified under the acceptance that humans have one body and will spend a lifetime learning the different stages and sensations that can be experienced within it. As a manual therapist, I use indicator muscle testing to prove to patients the potent power of their beliefs. We all love indisputable proof. I also use subjective responses (verbal feedback about changes felt) to invite both believers and nonbelievers alike to accept that something intelligent is happening within our tissues and that we have access to learning how to influence it.

Orthopedic or indicator muscle testing is my evaluation technique to select appropriate therapies for a person who struggles from a combination of physical and emotional discomfort. The physical and nonphysical portions of our bodies are no longer separate in my mind. Muscle testing helps patients gain trust in my ability to communicate with their symptoms and deeply hear their concerns. It has influenced my belief that with the right provider (truly an interpreter), everyone has access to learning the subtle language of the subconscious body. By adding this technique to your daily life, you may reveal issues that have stumped other doctors, guiding you to correct treatment plans.

Review Questions

1. Have you ever had a gut instinct that was so strong it physically affected you until you followed that intuitive guidance? Identify which area in your body was screaming the loudest to get the message across (for example, mind, stomach, chest).

2. Where does most of your information about alternative healing come from?

3. What style of self-learning do you subscribe to? Grade each from 1 to 5 (1 being your favorite, 5 least favorite):

   - reading self-help books and articles
   - visual/auditory—workshops, YouTube videos, or podcasts
   - verbal—word-of-mouth guidance from a trusted provider or loved one
   - tactile—an external source demonstrating on your body
   - sensory—experiencing internal benefits for yourself, then figuring out why

4. If you have tried an alternative healer:

   a. What was different about the communication style?
   b. Was their office environment comfortable or intimidating?
   c. How much time did they take to talk and get to know your experiences?
   d. What unexplainable sensation did you feel in your body during the care?
   e. Did anything make you uncomfortable? If so, was it your response / the work / the provider?

Whatever is flexible and flowing
will tend to grow.
Whatever is rigid and blocked will wither.
—Tao Te Ching

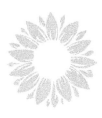

CHAPTER 4

Acupuncture and Becoming a Healer

Acupuncture and Becoming a Healer

A technique called *dry needling* has become popular within the sports therapy realm. The process involves a doctor using tiny needles to influence the muscles or nervous system without injecting anything into the body ("dry"). To the untrained eye, this intervention looks a lot like acupuncture. My local scope of practice in Oklahoma required one hundred hours of acupuncture training before being able to take a dry needling course or perform it on patients, so I registered for my first weekend course. Sitting in the dark basement underneath the loud adjusting tables of a busy chiropractic practice, I nervously glanced around at the collective of weirdos I was destined to spend many weekends with. I had a predetermined impression of the doctors who used the gift of acupuncture and the students who sought its abilities. I sneered at the testimonials, cringed at the ancient resources offered as research, and rolled my eyes as the clock refused to push on. Luckily, there were breaks with snacks every hour to look forward to.

On that first day, I used the mandatory time to study for other classes in school or read up on the latest self-help books, only glancing up if I heard the ancient teacher say something about multiple sclerosis or athletes. My heart always skips a beat when I hear a potential way to improve someone's discomfort with multiple sclerosis. MS is an autoimmune disease in which the myelin covering of the peripheral nervous system starts to break down and can no longer insulate the successful transfer of electricity throughout the body. Each case is different, but it traditionally creates stiffness in the body, hypersensitive skin, plaquing in the brain, and global immobility. My father suffers from a progressive version of the degenerative disease, and at the time, his accelerating symptoms in his right leg were a huge motivation to become the best doctor in the fastest way possible. Like many of the students around me, hidden underneath our ego, we learn medicine to take home and try to "fix" our families. We learn best by application, so if the material does not apply to our own body, we identify someone who does fit the condition to help it stick. Almost every medical student goes home excited to try a new exercise, diet, or manual therapy they learned on family members. And almost each of them comes back two weeks later disappointed, discouraged, or doubting their place in the field; the people you care most about are the hardest to help.

My father's version of MS affects his right leg, causing him to depend on the rest of his body to propel any movement. A slight limp progressed into occasional falls as we averted our gaze out of respect for his pride when he struggled to lift back up. Cane dependence eventually came, paired with welcome jokes and gifts of stylish walking pieces (one of which opened into a sword). I began chiropractic school around the time that his condition demanded a walker and wheelchair transportation outside the house. He is a kind and resilient man who chooses humorous love over complaining about his circumstances, and I wanted to be the one to help him make his miraculous recovery.

I aggressively offered lifestyle changes such as anti-inflammatory diets, meditation, supplements, and rehabilitation exercises, but breaking the cultural habits of your family is near impossible; just because you believe it does not guarantee someone else will receive benefits in the same way. It took a long time, but eventually he became curious about his daughter's doctor advice (notice the order). I adjusted my family as I learned each skill and was able to patch up small pains like a pinching shoulder, back spasm, or tight ribcage. But MS kept winning and I couldn't help but feel defeated by my lack of influence. Frustrated and scared that I could also succumb to the effects of the disease, I chose a defensive style of communication to prescribe the "right" way to heal at home. I didn't yet possess the subtlety of encouraging progress in others without condemning their previous behaviors and implying my parents' way of life was wrong. I am thankful for this bumpy road of combining work and homelife because it redirected my medical path toward less imposing techniques of healing. A harsh medical doctor who prescribes without empathy would never be enough. To help my dad—to help my patients and my own body—I would need to become a healer.

Healing Insight—Acupuncture and Meridian Therapy

In Traditional Chinese Medicine (TCM), there are considered to be three nervous systems: the voluntary network of systems that you choose to use, the involuntary autonomic system governed by the subconscious mind, and the acupuncture system of energetic channels in the body. Described as a flow of vital energies or qi (pronounced "chee"), the acupuncture system addresses the bioenergetic transmission between the client's magnetic field and an outside conductor of energy, such as the healer or the metal needles used. To connect and alter the energetic state of the body, tiny needles are placed in specific protocols along 361 points on the skin. Needling protocols along these points aim to improve electrical healing between twelve main channels of bioenergetic flow, called meridians. Each meridian is a vibrating line along the intangible body that is thought to coordinate with the characteristics of an organ system, offering the therapist information on its internal state of function. My medically trained brain struggled to comprehend how the twelve main channels could represent the

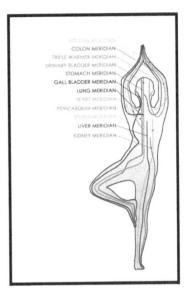

energy of organs such as the kidneys, lungs, intestines, stomach, and heart space. The main meridians are drawn in pairs, so when depicted, they do not come close to crossing the region of the organ they are named after. Were meridians of qi referral pain patterns initiated by visceral organ dysfunction?

I quickly learned that the energetic lines are not indicative of organ chemistry but are believed to be the creators of the emotions in which the brain manifests. For example, acupuncture philosophy finds that the gallbladder meridian creates and often stores a pool of emotions involving resentment, anger, and bitterness. A stagnant buildup of low-vibrational emotions within this organ causes stress and potential health issues if not balanced correctly. To resolve these imbalances, the emotional vibration can be restored through mental conversation so the brain encourages the organ to reset, or the meridian line is directly altered using needles to reset the communication that was triggering the brain to feel angry. New practitioners rely on the twelve main meridians with the rare addition of two special meridians known as the conception vessel and the governing vessel. The two midline meridians are large pathways that are believed to monitor and communicate with the smaller organ meridians that run through them. In energetic modalities, the governing vessel is also used to clear trapped emotions and stabilize the energetic body.[1] Reference *the Emotion Code* for more examples of how meridians help to clear trapped emotions.

An abnormal distribution of energy among these meridians is believed to disrupt the physical body all the way down to each vibrating cell. This continued disruption is thought to cause physiological imbalances, stagnant healing, and, if not resolved quickly, disease. Reports of chronic disorders such as asthma, infertility, stress, and musculoskeletal pain have been positively affected by acupuncturists in studied research. You can find an endless supply of such articles on PubMed.gov.

To apply the treatment, modern acupuncture tools are tiny stainless-steel needles with an average diameter the size of a strand of hair. Different metals are thought to create unique reactions, but stainless steel is the most commonly used in hopes of bringing imbalanced meridians back to a baseline of uniformed frequencies. Every system in our body, when vibrating and conducting as it's designed, will live in harmony or homeostasis. Excess production causes systematic turmoil and desensitization, while inhibited systems lead to organ failure which encourages systems to work harder to function. Acupuncturists are trained to recognize symptoms of physiological distress within the body and the specific needling patterns that resolve those issues. For example, a hyperactive thyroid will be cleared of emotional barriers during treatment so that the chemistry of the body can normalize its hormone production. If one acupuncture channel is blocked or malfunctioning, the energy will rise in other channels, potentially overriding them or putting them in excess. The metal needle is thought to bring any outliers of imbalanced measures back to a homeostatic baseline. Life is not sustainable without a balance of electric qi.

Some therapists, like myself, cannot memorize the endless combinations of all the acupuncture points, so they decide to utilize a more intuitive protocol of needling. Systems such as indicator muscle testing can direct the therapist where to needle. In addition to acupuncture needles, I use a *teishein* tool in my practice. This spring-loaded, non-piercing tool targets acupressure points without having to expose a vulnerable area of the body with a standard needle. The goal for the teishein, as well as all needling, is to transmit energy through the tool and reset the connection of electromagnetic flow along the skin. Less popular subdivisions of Chinese medicine include acupressure, tapping, cupping, or adding vibration to an acupuncture point. Using the hands as a medium, the electric relationship between the two bodies is utilized to realign the normal frequency of the targeted meridians.

Acupuncture within Manual Care

In Chinese medicine, the heart
is the seat of connection
between mind and body.
In yogic traditions, the heart is
literally and figuratively
our internal guide.
In western medicine, the heart
is a bundle of electrically
conductive tissue that governs us all.
— Baptise De Pepe

As a student learning this intangible acupuncture system, I had limited exposure to clinicians or patients who had tried this technique. I was defensively skeptical and had zero financial room to invest in any technique that wasn't medically respected or that would add to the already challenging title as an alternative health-care provider. I was reluctant to learn this system solely on the testimonials of strangers I met at an acupuncture seminar; surely, they were biased. I listened with an open mind but chose to implement my early applications in a physical, orthopedic style; I could absorb the physical component of needling that was accepted in the sports medicine and physical therapy world.

Dry needling (needles that don't inject anything into the skin) is great for sports injuries because the needle can alter trigger points or the fascia that surrounds muscle groups. Fascia is the innervated connective tissue that surrounds muscles, groups muscular lines of movement together, and alerts the brain about any pain experienced in the process. Just like the chakras in yoga, the lines of acupuncture's energy cannot be dissected or physically found in the body. Then in 2001, a licensed massage therapist published a groundbreaking textbook on the existence of fascial planes. His work demonstrates the relationship of dissected fascial planes, which are strikingly similar to the lines recognized as the meridians of acupuncture. Author Thomas Myers describes his theories of these correlating lines in his text *Anatomy Trains,* in which he uses the term *meridians* as longitude and latitude markers compared to the earth's geography—keeping the outlook strictly based on physical mechanics. I was amazed to read material that compared the mechanical component of fascial slings to the energetic experience of acupuncture meridians. In a structural way, fascial lines are "lines of pull," tissue lines that share tension, transmit strain, and stabilize bodily movements with rebound forces.[2]

Documented under ultrasound scans, an acupuncture needle has proven to create a spiral in the soft tissue below the skin. Somehow, the plain stainless-steel needles without any ribbing texture, twisted under the fingers of the provider, can grab the local tissue and spiral around the needle. This local hurricane shape is the component that initiates traction through the rest of the connecting layers.[3] The ultrasound in this study wasn't aimed at recording electromagnetic interference but instead focused on the effect of a twisted needle on subcutaneous tissue. Perhaps this fascial distortion from needling techniques will become a way to prove acupuncture's influence on distant parts of the body that were not touched by the provider during treatment.

Learning to Needle

I've found that chiropractors and physical therapists gladly utilize the intervention of acupuncture without wanting to learn the deep intention and connective philosophy that belongs with it. Although the students within my certification program were drawing meridian lines and memorizing their numbered points, we had no personal relationship with the treatment that the teachers asked us to believe in. I appreciate the importance of studying foundational skills such as meridian recognition, but I needed to witness results if I was going to advertise myself as a chiropractic acupuncturist.

At a rehabilitation seminar focused on jaw pain, the teacher introduced the class to dry needling to reduce temporomandibular joint dysfunction or TMJ. He gently guided the needle into the side of a student's jaw to release a trigger point in the lateral pterygoid muscle, one of the internal chewing muscles that is often a pain generator for TMJ issues. Viewing such precise treatment protocols reinforced my commitment to mastering the study of anatomy. Past memorizing pictures, digging through cadavers, and passing exams, this was the real work—where visual imagery from that study meets confident touch to deliver cool and calm healing hands.

Most of the students in class had the same expression on their face: *Did our first needling practice have to be on someone's face? Did he really expect us to do this after the demonstration?* Yes, yes, he did; a doctorate student truly is a guinea pig in a white coat. In small groups after the demonstration, it was my turn to be needled, and

I asked the teacher to be present to instruct the nervous student who was about to pierce my face. I asked, "What happens if we miss and hit the bone?"

"Here, I'll show you," he said while pushing my friend out of the way to jab my jawbone a few times. I prepared for pain but only felt a weird, deep pressure, like dentists warn you about after a numbing shot. He explained that the lining of the bone, known as periosteum, has fewer sensitive fibers than the surrounding soft tissue in response to mechanical stimulation. After surviving this demonstration, I relaxed, trusted my training, and learned amazing things the rest of the weekend.

Having this physical experience alongside the acupuncture training was a gift that allowed me to compare the benefits of each technique. The dry-needling technique is perfect for releasing trigger points and increasing local inflammation needed for healing. Although they aren't looking for it, I believe these providers are often influencing the meridians and emotional sites of pain while inserting needles. By the time my acupuncture course reached the needling portion of study, I was prepared to take my practice to the next level. I was taught a safe, comfortable way to needle that was much kinder than a "pistoning" or aggressive portion of the dry-needling technique. Acupuncture should be relatively pain-free; if the provider's intuition is correct, the body should welcome the needle gladly and without stressing the nervous system. My teacher, Pat Kahn, said it best when she explained that if the provider is gifted enough and in tune with the true cause of a patient's issue, "The best acupuncturist only needs one needle."

Between the Lines

When I finally became a doctor and had enough exposure to regular patients, I started to open my eyes to the confusing powers of acupuncture. With the right patient, I viewed the body as something deeper than inflamed muscles or immobile joints. I could feel changes in temperature at first while holding my hand over an injured area of the body. I allowed my visual creativity to guide my mind through layers of muscles, "seeing" the mechanical changes happening in the anatomical maze. Eventually, I could feel the electromagnetic pressure a few inches above the patient's body, and needles became the conductor between our two electrical systems. My hands learned to sense the heated meridians and could trace the buzzing resistance along the body until coming across a loss of connection, a blocked site of chi. If I moved too fast, the invisible pressure of the meridian line that pressed into my hand would disappear, as if falling off a track. A subtle shift back in line would reintroduce heat and pressure along the spiraling meridian.

The lines of pressure that I felt correlated with both systems. The tangible information followed the acupuncture meridian lines and the myofascial lines by Thomas Myers. For example, the muscles that I traditionally treat along the *deep front line* followed the same location and patterns of the acupuncture *liver meridian*. (See image 5.) Each fascial chain can be compared to one of the twelve main meridians.[2] Each musculoskeletal complaint that came in the office was treated as normal; align the body with chiropractic adjustments, address soft tissue imbalances and inflammation, and exercise new neurological patterns to train movement dysfunction. When pain lingered or the patient's goals were not met, I viewed the area of pain through the eyes of an acupuncturist and asked myself, "Which meridian line passes through this site of pain?" and "Which emotional trigger could have stirred this fascial chain to abort its normal function?" Once these two worlds collided within my treatment, I demonstrated this new paradigm to every patient who entrusted my healing hands with their progress.

After gaining their trust, I witnessed confusing experiences with their intelligent mind-body connection, confusion being the aftermath of panic-stricken. The first few times a needle refused to come out of the body, I blamed myself and my novice technique, nervously not letting the patient know that I was silently struggling. I had been trained to expect that the body will push a needle back out when it is done (even without movement or breathing pressure to encourage it), but I was not prepared for tissue to cling to a needle, preventing me from taking it out. Improper technique or aggressive movement while a needle is placed in the tissue can cause the shaft to bend, catching tissue layers and resisting a kind exit. But my technique was smooth, emotionally targeted, and noninvasive, so when this continued to happen, I was forced to believe in the unknown of healing. I learned to recognize that a "stuck" needle is a sign that the patient's emotional release was not done.

The mental imagery—or emotional conversation to rewrite a belief—needed more attention. After the healing mantra or correct metaphor was complete, the needle that I tugged on a moment before came out effortlessly. Patients could feel the difference between the resistance of an unfinished story and the ease of a closed emotional wound. They loved to see the magic of their own inner intelligence.

As it turns out, chiropractors have been influencing the meridian system without knowing it because when a spinal restriction is released, the acupuncture lines of associated points run right alongside the spinal segments. There are fourteen associated points in bilateral pairs along the spine, running on what is known as the bladder meridian. In addition to spinal adjustments, muscle testing can also offer an opportunity to witness physical progress after using the energetic system of acupuncture. Eastern medicine and AK practitioners, for example, combine indicator muscle testing with the meridian theory of acupuncture to ask the body about past trauma, stored emotions, and sites of trapped painful memories.[4]

If the muscle chosen to represent the chain goes weak after a stimulus or question, it is believed to answer as no. These weak chains are often contributing to unstable movement patterns, low back pain, pelvic floor incontinence, or TMJ issues. Once the physical body has been restored (adjust, stretch, rehab, etc.) with the intention to resolve that meridian muscle test, the indicator test is reapplied to show progress. Physical restrictions can alter the flow of electric impedance within the body that the acupuncture system aims to reconnect. Collagenous bands of scar tissue and joints that are out of optimal alignment are speculated to reduce the success of electric transmission in the body.[5] Acupuncture philosophy believes that emotions and resistant trauma memories can act as physical blockades as well.

Jackson's Unfinished Story

The longest fight I ever had with a needle that refused to come out was five minutes long, the longest five minutes of my career. I was tired and didn't want to address heavy emotions the day that Jackson came into my office with a spasm in his right shoulder blade. I had previously adjusted him and used soft tissue techniques without the success of permanently relieving his pain. In hopes of a superficial fix, I needled a trigger point in his infraspinatus muscle as we addressed the metaphor that often plagues this area, being "stabbed in the back." We used indicator muscle testing to discover if the original event was … Five years ago? *Super weak means no.* Ten years? *Weak means no.* Twenty? *Oh nice. A strong muscle. That's a yes.* The only trigger Jackson could think of during that time frame was that he and his younger brother started to fight more often around that age. I asked him to visualize forgiving his brother and what behaviors they both needed to demonstrate to heal that hurt, younger version of himself. Feeling satisfied and falling behind on my schedule, I went to pull the needle out and found zero give; a funnel of skin tented up to follow the lifting needle then recoiled back toward the shoulder blade when I let go.

I tried a few more times, making sure I did not twist the tissue too much and ruled out spinal restrictions along the superficial back arm line of fascia. Nothing. I am embarrassed to admit that I even used tweezers and my kinesiology scissors to try to pull the needle out. Again, nothing. I kept Jackson in the loop, so he knew I was having trouble with the needle, and he promised it wasn't hurting. I finally gave in and accepted my next patient would have to wait. I can't send a man out with a needle in his body! I calmed my mind and talked to him more about his brother's vantage point at that age. This conversation led to him revealing a trauma that he inflicted on his brother at that age. They had taken playing too far, and he had closed him in a box of some sort. His brother's annoyance turned into fear as Jackson scrambled to release his brother. Eventually, his brother was set free but obviously stressed for air, and it had shocked his body.

Jackson had held onto guilt for this mistake for many years and was projecting having sabotaged his brother's life onto his own body as punishment. Talking about the story as an adult allowed him to view it differently, make peace with young mistakes, and invited the young mental Jackson to return to his present state of adulthood. I was almost angry when the needle slid out of his shoulder effortlessly after our conversation. Jackson left that day without shoulder pain but with a true glimpse of how the intelligent body holds onto memories. I also recommended that he seek therapy for further discussion about the early trauma. I washed my face a few times before taking back the next patient, apologizing for the delay.

The Energy System of Acupuncture

A common complaint I hear during treatment sessions involves a pattern of sleep disturbance. Patients notice their body wakes them up at a certain point in the middle of the night, and it keeps happening. By reporting symptoms that spike at certain hours of the day or night, this offers a clinician information to categorize and identify the pain generator. Through Western medicine approaches, the doctor will rule out chemical variables that rise and fall depending on our circadian rhythm, such as cortisol or melatonin levels. Manual therapists will also make sure your body is comfortable in sleeping postures to alleviate sleep-disturbing pain. To an acupuncturist, persistent patterns of pain identify that an organ is experiencing emotional or energetic imbalances. Based on the "qi clock," organ behaviors have a peak hour of activity during a twenty-four-hour cycle. For example, most emotional pain wakes people up from 2:00 to 4:00 a.m., when the liver and lung meridians are most active. When the physical body sleeps, the subconscious mind is in control, relaying mental imagery in dreams with messages that we try to decipher in the morning. By addressing those meridian points, while the patient visualizes that time of night, the meridians can be cleared, and emotional trauma stirring in the subconscious mind can be brought to the surface.

In the energetic body, each of the meridians are thought to flow through governing regions known as the *dan tiens*. The dan tiens are regions of clustered qi where the energy within each meridian will travel through and communicate by. Depicted as the three main regions of energy grouping, the lower, middle, and upper Dan Tien are very similarly described like the chakras in yogic teaching—pools of energy that emanate from nerve plexuses within the physical body. Another parallel to yoga, Qigong is the practice affiliated with Chinese medicine that aims to cultivate and balance inner energy levels through intentional movement. Most modern yoga practitioners don't realize that this intention lies beneath their glamorous physical practice. If you have never seen the flow of Qigong, look it up on YouTube and get mesmerized by the fluid practice of a centered mind-body.

Know Your Elemental Behavior

One of the most enticing portions of the acupuncture system is how a traditional practitioner categorizes a patient's body or personality to fit into one of the five elements in Traditional Chinese Medicine. Earth, metal, water, wood, and fire are the five elements of TCM that are thought to govern specific organ systems. Acupuncturists often reference an elemental chart (see image 6) to witness the connecting relationship between organ systems and

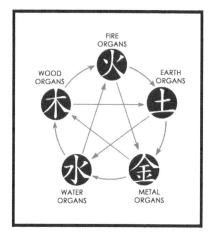

then quickly identify important needling points for each condition. The Kho cycle (the star in the center) is designed to depict the laws of destruction between the five elements; wood destroys earth by breaking up the soil, earth destroys water by confining it to a space, water destroys fire by extinguishing it to find equilibrium, fire destroys metal by melting it, and metal destroys wood by cutting it.

Each element is a representation of two to four organs. The circle that surrounds the Kho cycle depicts how the energy of each element or organ system complements the subsequent group. Using these metaphors or pulse diagnostics, the acupuncturist will analyze the organ system that needs energetic relief as well as which organ system is responsible for overpowering it to perform poorly.

The categories of a patient's build and personality helps the healer alter their care to compliment the needs of their elemental patient. If a very strong patient comes into my office with a highly inflamed body and uses intense words to describe their pain, I notice a fiery behavior and implement water-focused care to subside the temperament. Using fluid massage, cooling oils, and continuous movement, I guide their acupuncture system and nervous system back to a contained flame. Or another example, if a very thin-framed woman comes into my office with reported brain fogginess and migraines, I assume her airy temperament needs to be grounded and to have her internal pressure system stabilized. I will guide her with breath to reset the pressure in her head, playing to her strengths, instead of being forceful on her joints or adding a lot of weight to her body during adjustments. Ultimately, these elements remind the healer to be mindful of how to communicate and approach each unique intervention. In acupuncture, we will either match the elemental behavior of the patient or try to complement it when it is out of balance. Using this concept at home, can you recognize when a child's extreme mood can be balanced by using a complementary language, color, or temperature? When looking through the lens of TCM, we can apply its philosophies into many aspects of our daily lives, such as the home practice of feng shui, which is also governed by the five elements of balance.

Paul's Skyfall

> Some treatments repair the body in a way
> the body could not induce alone,
> other treatments merely enlist
> the mind's potent power
> to optimize the health of the body.
> — Lisa Rankin, MD

Acupuncture is not recommended to use as a diagnostic tool, due to low measure of reliability and ability to recreate protocols within research, but it is an amazing tool to teach a provider to read the responses of a patient's body, which in return offers more information about the effects of a condition. With the increase of both observation and tactile skills, better diagnostic questions are addressed. The more questions that we intuitively ask, the more subjective clues the patient will provide. This subtle part of the pain story can be a vital piece of the puzzle that the patient would not have affiliated with the condition. One such case was with a patient named Paul. He came into my office complaining of very sharp pain at the base of one side of his neck that had been progressively advancing for two weeks. He assumed it was from his workouts at the gym.

When looking up, a debilitating "zing" shot from his upper trapezius muscle into his lower cervical spine. I used all my normal approaches for this common pain, such as cervical and thoracic spine adjustments, soft tissue care for muscles in spasm, breath restoration, and cupping to decompress the upper trapezius. Although his pain subsided by the end of the first visit, it was obvious that he still had limited range of motion and was fearful to test the neck's limits. A few visits passed by, and I threw all I could at him; still, the pain relief only lasted a few days following each session. Eventually, I addressed the emotional component of his pain and ran my acupuncture protocol over his symptoms. Heat in the neck, inability to look up … As the words ran through my mind and my hands massaged his upper trapezius muscle, I got a quick image in my mind of him falling. Swallowing my pride, I chose to trust my intuition and ask about any recent falls or bad dreams potentially. He answered no, so I moved forward with the needling portion of acupuncture treatment, shrugging off my overactive imagination.

Back to business, I placed one needle deep into his upper trapezius, angled away from the lung apex and important vessels close to the region. In previous chapters, I described how cellular memory is built into the tissue that was utilized for certain movements; the tissues learn how to replicate and respond to movement. On the surface, I can trigger the memory, response, and emotional release of most fascial movements, but some of the deeper layers cannot be influenced without a portal; an acupuncture needle is my favorite portal. The needle that I was slowly guiding into Paul's muscle finally touched a resistant tissue of a trigger point when he blurted out, "Wait! I went skydiving!"

"When did you do that?" I asked.

"Two weeks ago," he said, laughing in disbelief. We left the needle in the tissue to maintain a connection with the "trapped" emotional layer as we discussed his motives for skydiving. By using visual meditations and a few prompt questions for self-inquiry, he was able to decide that, just like his life, his body wasn't losing control, and he would no longer throw himself into extremes to prove it.

After sitting up, Paul looked up to the top of the room with barely any pain left in his neck. The unhealthy motivation that drove him to go skydiving was the barrier we needed to heal before pain relief would stick. And it did. With maybe one or two fine-tuning sessions to prevent a relapse in pain, Paul was introduced to a new lifestyle and way to view his emotionally fluent body. I have had the pleasure of discussing his journey through awareness over the following years during sporadic treatment visits.

Becoming a More Evolved Healer

The medicine you have to offer
is often the medicine that you need.
— Julia Plevin, *The Healing Magic of Forest Bathing*

Acupuncture was the first of many training certifications I would elect to study outside of chiropractic school's curriculum. Its influence grew like a rolling snowball; the more I used it, the more I trusted it and witnessed positive results. When I felt brave enough to advertise offering acupuncture as a service, I found colleagues and people within my community who regularly use its techniques in addition to traditional health care. Years after completing my acupuncture training, when I opened my old binders for inspiration to write this chapter, I found a torn-out page, folded in the front pocket, that I apparently used as a gum wrapper during a weekend course. The visible words that were not creased over belonged to a list of recommended ways to become a more evolved healer—a word that obviously held little weight at that time in my professional journey. At that robotic stage of being a student, I couldn't afford (financially and academically) to heal using intuition or admit to believing in our ability to influence energetic fields in the body; I had to answer questions correctly and pass the exams that people with different beliefs had created years before. I was still fighting an invisible enemy to prove that *chiropractor* was a respectable title, let alone *healer.* I gave my less evolved self some grace and understood that she couldn't appreciate other views of healing that didn't align with Western traditions until having a physical experience of her own. *She will,* I thought as I glanced through the list and thought about my first acupuncture session:

Lying on a warm, cloth-covered table in Kansas City, I met with a lovely woman who I found from a Google search with good reviews and reasonable prices. This tiny Chinese woman would make me a believer, regardless of fitting the acupuncture stereotype perfectly. As she covered my body with intentionally placed needles, she asked me normal questions about my reported hip pain and hormone disruptions. After I survived the needling process, I finally relaxed into treatment and fought off sleep for the next fifteen minutes. I occasionally snuck open an eye to peek at her curious movements of fluid hand swiping, air pushing, and palm pulsing above the needles that lined my body. A palpable heat rose in my stomach when her hand covered the area and then, as if she had magnets in hand, guided the heat from head to toe. The original description I developed that day to explain the shifting and settling sensations inside my body is the same one I use today to give patients a visual understanding of how needling releases fascial adhesions. Remember the unlocking vault door in Gringott's Bank that catapulted into motion underneath the floating hand of the banker? That was my body under her magnetic touch.

Her flowing treatment stopped as I felt the heat settle into my right hip crease, the area of pain that I planned to use to test the effectiveness of acupuncture. She broke the silence saying, "In my head, I can visualize tubes being pulled out of your body and a battle with infection. In your paperwork, you mentioned having hip surgery. Were there infectious complications?" I looked up from the table, assuming she was looking at my hip surgery scar on my leg, only to find that she had stopped over one of my invisible appendectomy scars about a foot higher up; she knew I had laparoscopic surgery to fight a septic appendix without any history beyond my musculoskeletal reports of soccer injuries. Shocked and embarrassed that I had not mentioned it before, I told her about my appendix that had basically shriveled up and died during one of my seasons in college. In a patient way, she explained how the body, especially scars, stores an imprint of the physical and emotional memories that we experience at the time of an invasive procedure. She recommended I start a personal routine of scar tissue massage, deep breathing underneath the site of the scar, and to focus my studies on the mentality of injuries. Based on the tears that were coming out of my eyes and the relief in hip tension that was present only moments before, I was easy to convince.

By sharing this guide, I can offer a catalog of success stories that I witnessed behind the closed doors of an office. Underneath healing hands, the philosophies of chiropractic, muscle testing, and acupuncture worked their magic. When applied in a safe and appropriate way, I was able to learn a system that combined sports chiropractic with the energetic themes of these practices.

East meets West on my table, and I often joke while teaching workshops that "acupuncture was my gateway drug into the weird world of energetic health care." By applying Western manual therapies to the problematic region, pain melted away, emotions were expressed, the meridian's electric circuit could flow once more, and patients were open to developing a higher consciousness for all outlets of life. As stated in Dr. Richard Yennie's acupuncture training:

How to become a more evolved healer:

1. Connectedness
2. Transformation process
3. Removing blockages to healing
4. Content with detachment
5. Future vision
6. Gratitude and surrender

Connectedness

In my third year of practice, I was asked to present a lecture to the female students at a chiropractic university to help inspire them and improve their adjusting skills. The adjusting skills that I focused on for most of the seminar were not the actual "crack" of a cavitating manipulation. I helped these women remember that their ability to connect with patients should be effortless and perhaps easier than their male colleagues' approach. Connection sounds simple. Plug in the cord, type in the right Wi-Fi password, or physically sit across from a woman who reached out to you on social media to network. There are many layers of connection. In medicine and healing arts, many providers lose that ability to see the person they are working on. Obviously, they see the patient, hear the conversation, and interact enough to create a care plan and diagnose an intervention. But that is the most surface level of healing we have access to. The doctor could accomplish those same tasks easily while still thinking about fantasy football, what fight they had last night with their spouse, or what relative the patient reminds them of from their past.

Presence defines our ability to connect. Full presence is a gift that few of us truly get to experience. You will know when it's happening. There is a magic that we can't explain that happens when the eyes listen, facial gestures are approachable, body language is inviting, and touch is respectful yet supportive. To be an evolved healer is to be an evolved human, weightless from emotional fear or internal turmoil that clouds every hour of our high-functioning day. In my mind, a clinician or practitioner is a very qualified person who sees a patient as a body, a paycheck, an insurance liability, and a challenge. In medicine and healing arts, many providers lose that ability to see the person they are working on. A healer can be a person who respects medical bylaws; they witness aspects of the healthcare field and respect them but then choose to go deeper. A healer looks at the whole human experience and trusts the interconnection between emotions, perceptions, environment, and their resulting physical symptoms. A healer views the person in front of them as a cosmic delivery; the universe perfectly aligned the two of you to meet— on this time and day—for a greater purpose than either party may understand for years to come.

Transformation Process

We all have a body and a fierce need to understand its capabilities while creating life around it. As the patient, find a practitioner in all fields who supplies you with those values; you have that right to shop around until the right healer comes along. Then watch the magic happen! Trust your doctors and health-care providers but learn for yourself what intelligence you already have within you. No outside source can offer you permission to access what you already feel and accomplish inside each day. We are here to help you understand it, connect you with your goals, jump-start a healing process, and lead you down a path toward self-care.

As the practitioner, you'll know you're making the transition from clinician to a healer when you start to witness yourself in every person who sits on your table. Professional boundaries are maintained, but universal boundaries start to blend as you are now able to relate to almost anyone you treat. Instead of viewing their predicament or form of expression as separate from your own experiences, you'll hear the answers to your own life in their epiphanies. Intentional connection with your work is the first step towards changing apathy into sympathy. Deep sympathy transforms into empathy and ignites a call to action for the responsible provider. With this recognition, you will start using more loving words, high-vibrational techniques, and inviting approaches to guarantee that people are heading in the right direction (whether that includes your services or not).

Removing Blockages to Healing

A healer sets the scene. The room that they treat in is a personal sanctuary and their bedside manner is taken to the next level. Every detail has been taken into account to make the person who walks in the door comfortable—temperature, adaptable lighting, soothing colors on the walls and on the provider's clothes, the volume at which they speak, the height at which the healer stands in comparison to the patient, and so on. Where the doctor stands can make or break someone's comfort levels; permission is always acquired before touching (regardless of the region). These extra efforts are not time-consuming, and they create a lifestyle that is second nature to a healer.

One major trait of the recently awakened healer is their ability to help patients feel and witness the now. I am sure you've heard of terms such as grounding and mindfulness, which are both included in a variety of practices that help our anxious minds focus on a present experience. All humans heal better when in a fully present, connected state of mind in which we feel safe, heard, and supported by the people we entrust our health with. To guide someone to be in the now, the provider should aim to pull their fears back from the thought of an injury becoming permanent or that a symptom is a small surface sign of some threatening pathology underneath. As the trusted clinician or healer, use your skill set to show each patient how to express their current sensations, devoid of tacking futuristic fears onto the experience.

A healer helps their patients develop an empowered partnership in which they acknowledge their own ability to create healthy self-perceptions and lifestyle habits. This gives each patient a sense of control that their current decisions will precede a healthy future. The late yoga instructor BKS Iyengar once stated, "The brain is the hardest part of the body to adjust." A skewed mental perception of pain can be a large blockage to permanent healing. Excavating the layers of trauma in a person's life is a long process and won't always fall under the provider's scope of practice. For chiropractors or body workers, refer to the appropriate therapy but then try to offer day-one relief, meaning use a combination of manual therapies with empathetic interactions to help patients witness empowering changes and to offer incremental hope for what's to come. Using the tools above to reduce mental resistance to receiving care will benefit both the patient and the confidence of the provider.

I often hear new patients explain that they left their previous doctor because they felt that the care was mindless, repetitive, and fear provoking. Even if their previous chiropractor was doing the same manual work that I do, they delivered it in a way that made the patient subconsciously close off from its benefits. Removing blockages to healing is in my mind, the most important role of chiropractors, acupuncturists, and bodyworkers. Aligned bodies with even tone can communicate thoughts, movement, and system regulation effortlessly.

For providers, if you have heard the little voice in the back of your mind ask why the patient's body is not naturally restoring and maintaining their own function, then congratulations, you are becoming a healer. You are starting to look beyond the comforts of a routine adjustment or quick service and beginning to trust that your business will adjust accordingly if you decide to spend more time with each patient. You can empower an educated, high-functioning patient and be successful at the same time. Have faith that when healed people are released from care, they will refer their loved ones to you and continue the never-ending flow of humans seeking relief from a gifted healer.

Content with Detachment

Detaching from unrealistic identities as a health-care provider frees up space to allow new learning and interests to fill the void of a struggling business or an unfulfilling niche. A young chiropractic practice demands an identity—a new persona that you must fully engulf to attract like-minded patients. "If you like golf, be the best golf doctor there is." "If you want to treat CrossFit patients in your town, then join a gym and integrate yourself into the community as soon as you move there." Advice from mentors and management companies suggest new clothes and personalities that will surely create the face of a promising business.

After moving to Tulsa, I surrendered to the call and registered to take six months of a two-hundred-hour yoga teacher training. With hopes that this would further develop my growing personal practice and become my niche, I selected a program that was outside the Tulsa city limits. Two hours away, I could be vulnerable and learn around strangers without having to satisfy the personal depiction of Dr. Marina that I kept up with in Tulsa. Potential patients were everywhere, right? It was this mindset that prevented me from moving forward in both professional and personal relationships for the rest of the year. The ego of

Dr. Marina was the first and only thing I'd have to drop to successfully join the women in my program and offer my best to the Tulsa community.

My time in teacher training helped me approach some uncomfortable expectations I had for being a chiropractor and, more importantly, that being a chiropractor did not need to define me. There are countless reasons that the body can catapult into dis-ease outside the areas that my skill set and manual training can resolve. Sometimes, the mechanism of pain calls for care that doesn't include your help. Learning that you are not for everyone is a hard pill to swallow as a young doctor. Yoga training helped me to accept this truth and by doing so, allowed my perception of care to broaden, encouraging me to treat patients as more than a chiropractor alone. I was one person meeting another person each visit. I still wonder about my earliest patients, wishing I could go back and deliver my better formed message and clinical interventions. I can only hope they found another source of alternative care and didn't lose hope after one or two underwhelming visits with my less evolved self.

A healer recognizes that in a treatment session, they are not the priority. Each visit is an opportunity to do your best work without expecting a thank you or compliment afterwards. Sometimes the purpose of our best efforts is to help others realize their own. Drop the ego and listen, so that when the patient reports no change in pain after one hour of grueling care, you have enough information to demonstrate their progress in movement, breath retention, range of motion, or overall emotional well-being. Although the product of removing pain can become addicting, those results do not validate your time or efforts spent.

Gratitude and Surrender

Intention dictates what each healer will find. I never planned to join a medical sports practice and become exposed to the unknown depths of our mind-body, but as anyone who touches—deeply touches—bodies for a living can attest, unexplainable things are bound to happen on the table. Unanswered and unknown feats of the human spirit will compel all new doctors to question what is truly at play inside us. I believe that the reason more doctors and health-care providers don't open their minds to the idea of invisible intelligence is because once the veil is lifted and they witness the unknown, what are they supposed to do about it?

It is overwhelming to try to solve all of life's issues in a short treatment. It is also terrifying to think you are not doing enough for every patient in a career where you already offer so much of yourself (sometimes too much). Feeling like you're falling behind the clinical times and that your colleagues have access to information that you don't is crippling. The only words of comfort that I can offer to those struggling in between the world of healing or clinical treating is that we are meant to experience both healing and learning in seasons. Not every day of practice is going to be legendary or lifesaving. Some months, clinicians are fired up to trial new learning techniques, and then they fall into a healing rhythm until the urge for new learning comes back to the surface. Depending on where we are in our own personal journey with physical, mental, emotional, and spiritual health, those external factors will dictate whether we are safely prepared to move forward within our work.

Turmoil at home creates turmoil in our careers and vice versa. Surrendering to a deeper level of conscious healing takes having foundational areas of life in place first, a surprisingly cyclic and regenerating list of needs. For the struggling licensed healers and self-healers, keep trying to surrender to the unknown. Continue to seek out ways to learn, reinspire, and reaffirm your original choice of leading a life dedicated to helping others heal. In my world of combined philosophies, I have witnessed people healing themselves without chiropractic, without medicine, and without a doctor guiding every decision. Refrain from letting another person with a different healing style belittle your own. We all subscribe to the practices and behaviors that suit our current goals or desires. Don't let someone else's beliefs make you question the success that you've already accomplished.

Open-Minded, Future Vision

During a yoga retreat in the hills of the Ozarks, I was introduced to a very easy way to demonstrate layers of perception. I now use this technique to help people with panic attacks pull their tunnel vision back to a normal visual depth. This exercise demonstrates a calming way to expand your reality so that it may include the healing techniques that your body deserves. It can be done with many of the senses, such as hearing or physical touch, but the visual version is my favorite:

Layers Exercise

Sit outside where your field of vision isn't obstructed by a cubicle or a whiteboard. Hold your hand at an arm's length with the palm facing away from you, about the height of your forward gaze. Without moving your hand or eyes, notice the subtle layers of depth that your eyes can focus on, without changing the lens. The fingers seem close, but what is just beyond that, and behind that, and surrounding that? Zoom out in layers until you've hit your eyes capacity, then, zoom back in towards your hand one layer at a time.

The way our brain draws our attention to priorities is determined by our reality, a view of the world as an accumulation of our experiences, beliefs, and motives (more on this in chapter 8). If you want to see only fingers as broken or not broken, your brain will never distract you with the endless void of sounds and images behind your target. With an open mind and trust that we can handle the massive amount of information that lies beyond, our blinders open and give us a larger chance to see.

For healers, see what is creating the superficial symptoms, see what is truly bothering this human on your table, see what trust they are placing in you to be their advocate for healthy changes. What priority issue is creating the superficial symptoms that we repetitively treat and chase? We won't always know the true answer, but at least we are one step closer to the solution than those who are not asking the hard questions.

For those of you who feel disconnected from the call within this list as if it only speaks to healers or providers, I want you to unveil your own gifts and apply all the concepts into your own realm of a career or household role. Mothers and fathers are unsung heroes and healers; each day, you are challenged with observing unspoken signs of physical discomfort and emotional development. Using the gifts to become a more connected healer, you may learn to understand and potentially harness the subtle dialect that your body already uses to interact with your family or coworkers. We all need a reminder to empathetically listen, without the intent to answer. Allow room for personal interpretation of this list because your life views and beliefs will fill in the blanks. The inalienable gift of healing that we all possess calls for less resistance and more connection.

Review Questions

1. Thinking about interactions with your medical provider (alternative or not):

    a. Did you feel invited to participate in the direction of care and outcomes?

    b. Was the environment welcoming to questions, concerns, and voiced goals?

2. If negative memories come up, how has that experience altered your health care utilization?

    a. Could you have better worded your needs and taken control of the interactions?

    b. Is there someone who could have helped improve the situation by being there?

3. Do you view medical providers as a sign of hope or authority?

4. Who do you currently believe has the final say when it comes to altering your body? Has that been different in the past?

5. Can you remember a time you sought a second opinion from a gut instinct that proved correct? Can you remember that empowering feeling of understanding your body?

6. Send gratitude to any provider who has ever offered you the chance to improve your outlook on health and personal abilities, who created a safe scene for your body to do what it does best—adapt and heal.

7. For clinicians, where is there room in your current practice to expand your techniques to include more intuitive protocols?

   a. Do you long to work for someone who allows you to be creative and autonomous?

   b. What identities or fears do you anticipate struggling with while transforming your style of practice?

   c. If you could talk to yourself in five years to ask how practice is going, what would you want to know specifically?

If you want to find the secrets of the universe,
think in terms of energy,
frequency, and vibration.
— Nikola Tesla

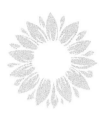

CHAPTER 5

Quantum Healing

Healing Insight—Quantum Physics in the Body

Quantum physics is the study of subatomic particles and their interactive behaviors within the universe. In this field of physics, we are asked to learn beyond the comforts of Newton's predictable outcomes, limited possibilities, and the material measurements that are taught in school. Stepping out of that 3-D mindset into the unknown, limitless world of quantum is confusing at first and may not seem to apply to anyone who isn't an astrophysicist. But the visibility of this field, and the terminology itself, is making its way into mainstream attention outside of an academic world. Popular movies, TV shows, and countless books are using the rising trend to lightly educate our society on quantum's existing theories and its involvement in a limitless future. Most directors and writers use this branch of science to fill the void that our current technology can't explain within their storylines. To quote the actor Paul Rudd in *Ant Man 2,* "Do you guys just put the word *quantum* in front of everything?" Well, yes. Yes they do, Paul.

Even within the growing field of intuitive health-care providers, I've heard the word *quantum* used as an umbrella term to explain physical experiences that can't be comprehended. For the purposes of this chapter, I want to expose health-conscious readers and health-care providers to the paradigm of a quantum reality in relation to the human body. It is an ever-advancing field, and I do not claim to be an expert, but if my introduction to the field ignites a new way to view your vibrationally active body and its healing capabilities, my work will be done.

In an effort to explain how everything is connected (immaterial matter and every living species in between), the accepted mathematics of quantum physics suggests that the answers to our vast and unknown universe may be solved by looking closer at the tiny building blocks of life. More importantly, looking at the space in between them. Living cells consist of atoms, atoms that are built by a varying number of electrons, protons, neutrons, and something unique to quantum physics, an even smaller subatomic particle called a quark. By learning that the universe is made up of energetic particles, we embrace the invisible existence of an electromagnetic field. A traditional depiction within an atom shows how electrons circle the nucleus in an electromagnetic orbit because their negative charge respects the limits of a positively charged nucleus, creating magnetism. In relation to the electron, an electromagnetic field is so large that it looks like 99.999 percent empty space, but that space is actually filled with energy and frequencies.[1] These tiny electromagnetic units are the building blocks of everything we encounter on Earth.

The ordinary matter of the world that we live in is made up of elements from the periodic table, which, is only 5 percent of the total energy of the universe. According to NASA, outside of that periodic table, 68 percent of the universe consists of dark energy, not matter. Coined *dark matter* due to its behavior of avoiding light interactions, the particles within that 68 percent hide from the light spectrum.[2] Humans can only visualize colors and frequencies that make up less than 1 percent of all the light spectrum of electromagnetic frequencies, so almost every living mass that we interact with, at its smallest components, is in constant motion beyond what the eye can see.

Scientists and theoretical physicists have been working on improving our understanding of wavelike energy since the seventeenth century. It was historic physicist Max Planck who originally believed that energy wasn't continuous as previously taught. In the early 1900s, he discovered that energy is "quantized" into tiny energy packets. In the quantum theory of matter (sorry, Paul), energy is considered to lump together in temporary particles that continuously form and disappear; both ordinary and dark matter demonstrate clusters like this. Together, clusters form energetic fields that become the foundational building blocks of living organisms. Planck was also vital in discovering the existence of photons, a massless particle that moves at the speed of light within an electromagnetic field. A photon is a quantum, or primary particle of light.

These advances collaborated with the work of other bright minds such as Bohr, Einstein, De Broglie, and then in the seventies, John Wheeler. Each breakthrough expands upon the existing beliefs of previous experts and continues to mold our modern view of an ethereal source that doesn't seem to want to be tied down. Like most quantum physicists, Wheeler viewed the microscopic universe as an intelligent source that avoided predictable outcomes of classical mechanics. He believed that humans had the ability to influence the particles of matter by simply observing them due to the famous double slit experiment. Wheeler's thought experiments aimed to understand why photon particles behave erratically during testing and refuse to demonstrate fixed results while the experiment was observed. Before technological advances, the open-ended results made space to question if intelligent matter is influenced or directed by our intentions. Now that the classic experiment has been modernized, physicists have found that the outcome of a traveling photons (and electrons) can act as both particles and waves.

Despite the challenge of tracking light particles, we know that photons are reeled into stability when absorbed by atomic molecules. These molecules can transfer the photon energy or keep the upgrade to maintain its collective field. The interdependent particles in an electromagnetic field are held together by a perfectly balanced electromagnetism that represents the successful coordination between internal and external environments of each primary unit. The units are stable and responsive, as if beads could be strung on an invisible guitar string, a pluck of the string would send the tiny particles into waves of vibrating frequencies. This motion is an adaptation method. In response to stimulants of the world, frequencies can alter matter to generate the reactions of life. A hand, for example, to the eye looks solid and formed. Through the eyes of quantum physics, imagine zooming into the deep layers of the tissues that make up a hand to visualize how a mass made of living tissue is in constant motion—constantly healing, replenishing, and growing.

On estimate, there are roughly thirty-seven trillion cells in the body that dance around according to the laws of our personal electric system and the external laws of an electromagnetic atmosphere. Each living cell balances its own tiny environment while coordinating with the success of the larger ecosystem. Individual cells lump together to make the tissues that build organs and organ systems. The organ systems are then controlled by the nervous system—the master system of the human body—that alerts you when homeostasis is compromised and it's time to seek a guide from the health-care system.

Taking Off the Whitecoat

Author and researcher Joe Dispenza explains that quantum physics tells us that our environment is an extension of our mind and that by recognizing our ability to influence a greater field of energy, we begin to bond within a quantum field of intelligence, "beyond space or time." What does that mean? To me, he is artistically describing how our acceptance of the unknown that exists beyond our awareness is a major stepping-stone that each person will make at a separate time in life. It is the ah-ha moment where we connect the electrical circuit within our body to an external causation of electricity. We are a collection of electrical transducers; our senses convert energy through sound, sight, and smells into another form of energy that the brain then interprets. Once we are each introduced to invisible possibilities, maybe even catch a glimpse of a personal physical experience, we'll enter a paradigm of awareness that cannot be forgotten.

In 2018, the year that I dove into this confusing world of intuitive medicine, a mentor of mine told me to stop identifying with the search to become content within my craft. "I don't like that word for you," he said over Skype one day. "It's no use. You'll never be content on the path you're trying to take. You love to learn, grow, and challenge the constricts of traditional health-care norms." He was right. I studied hard and became a chiropractor with a flair for the arts. Music made more sense to me than technology, speaking in front of an audience gave me more satisfaction than a crisp joint cavitation ever could, and I too easily got lost in the unspoken words of bodies to listen to the rules that confine healers. That's the danger of wishing to be content; it promises finality, that you've arrived. As an intuitive health-care provider, I wasn't ready to arrive until I had the necessary gifts that would enable me to bring others into that space. Aristotle defined wisdom as intuitive reason combined with scientific action. I was experiencing the intuition and the confusing results, but I didn't have the science to back it up and to present as wisdom. Thus began my journey into researching quantum physics and quantum healing.

What Is Quantum Healing?

Since that realization in 2018, I've devoted my practice to demonstrating how intuitive care and intentional healing can scientifically alter the body. Quantum healing is an intriguing topic that helped me sleep at night until I learned to trust that I can help others without always having a *why* or definition of *how*. As a healing modality, energetic bodyworkers believe that quantum physics is the key to explaining how our transferred electricity or shared energy can alter the body of a patient.[3] One familiar law within physics states that energy can neither be created nor destroyed; it can only change forms. Instead of blindly memorizing this rule for a test in high school, let's apply it to a life of energetic medicine. Through the intention of a sensitive and trained provider, quantum healing focuses on giving the body back its energy balance in order to facilitate healing without having to resort to medical interventions such as surgery or medications. I've found that most people are open to the fact that we constantly combine fields with other people throughout the day and maybe have heard that the heart alone can create an electromagnetic field measurable in a ten-foot radius around the body.[4] But those same individuals need more proof to support the notion that humans could have an ability to influence it through mental intention.

Quantum energy healing is based on the principle that a healthy, high-vibrational electromagnetic frequency (EMF) can positively benefit the living tissue it is directed toward. Supporters believe that to facilitate healing, the body must be in mental, physical, and spiritual balance, delivered by healthy vibrations. Recalling the study from the *Journal of Integrative Sciences* in 2015, researchers found that plants thrive in an environment of good music compared to a struggling plant that has been in constant contact with violent or "bad" music. The team reported that sound waves accelerated the synthesis of cellular metabolism in plants and promoted better growth.[5] Plants also behaved differently to different music types and frequency; "the notes are designed on the basis of the quantum vibrations that affect the plant at the molecular level." Remember how many cells we have? Let's feed them well with good vibrations.

Good Vibrations

Have you ever heard a monk bellow a loud, long chant in a movie? In yoga classes, a common chant of *om* is sung to unify the group intention. The chant sounds like *ohhhhhmmmmm* and is drawn to look like a "3.0" symbol, which depicts the three separate sounds that create the total effect: a, u, m. The three sounds of the chant blend together and collectively vibrate at a frequency of 432 Hz, which is speculated to be the same frequency as everything in nature, a great collective of vibration. There are many scientific studies aimed at disproving the om frequency, but small sample sizes have found health markers of decreased respiratory rate, heart rate, and blood pressure while listening to music tuned to this frequency.[6]

Why could its relevance affect the body? The body is a collaboration of different molecules that each follow their own laws of vibration. Each molecule, tissue, and organ will be influenced by large frequencies that come from governing systems or external forces. Just like the collective product of the three-part om frequency, our body is a compilation of countless frequencies that produce a final product. That product, if made of mostly healthy and high-vibrational frequencies, will thrive and adapt well to the stressors of life. If the final product is built of mostly low frequencies due to poorly functioning systems and stagnant regulation, the body will live in an environment of stress, vulnerability, and survival. If you want to dig, the internet offers an endless source of frequency levels from living systems in the body, to plants, planets, crystals, and emotional states. It helps to compare vibrations levels of things that are relatable to grasp the concept.

High-vibrational readings denote quickly moving frequencies, an increase of repetitive stimulation, and greater influence. Low-vibrational frequencies suggest long wavelengths, limited influence, and slower stimulation. Generally low-vibrational sources are related to unhealthy, non-life-sustaining frequencies. The world around us is a melting pot of frequencies, some of which we know how to alter. For most of us, trying to wrap our head around the frequency of Earth (the Schumann resonance of about 430.65 Hz) or the frequency of the heart (1–2 Hz) is complicated to relate to, but hearing a variety in musical frequencies is easy to differentiate.

The "do, re, mi" scale is a recognizable method that names an ascending scale of notes. Each note is assigned a frequency. The "do" of this scale is usually sung as the note C. Depending which C you pick on the piano to start, each octave has a different-sounding C, with appropriately altered measurements of frequency. On a piano, when middle C is struck, the key shocks a cord, which then vibrates in the back of the instrument at 261.625 Hz, producing a sound. The lowest C note toward the far left of the piano comes in ringing at 32.7 Hz. Which tone gives the impression of a happy note? The higher one! Most dark and ominous scores utilize low note combinations and chords to influence the listener's mood. We have our own unique acoustic mechanics built into the body, and when we reproduce a note to match an accompanying instrument, we internally buzz to project an external frequency into space.

Author of *The Healing Code*, Alex Lloyd, claims, "It all comes down to physics, since everything ultimately exists as its most common denominator: energy, with a corresponding vibrational frequency. Any frequency can be changed if we only know how to do so." If every living cell has its own charge, then all plants, all animals, all elemental building blocks have electricity. By being connected at the core, we collectively exist and vibrate in the same energy field. Our collection of frequencies may be different, so we have different experiences, but at the core of physics, we are all the same.

Many health-care providers use an EMF assessment to complement their own clinical expertise (chiropractors, acupuncturists, osteopaths, physical therapists, massage therapists, counselors). Other alternative energy-healing practices, such as reiki and sound healing, utilize this vibrational approach to connect the provider and patient. The vitality of quantum energy healing, similarly to chiropractic, believes that the human body has the natural ability to heal itself; sometimes it just needs to be rebooted and guided back to its natural state of peace.

Quantum Healing under the Microscope

Spiritual author and front runner in the field of energy medicine Deepak Chopra describes that quantum healing is a method that "moves away from external, high-technology methods toward the deepest core of the mind-body system." During his clinical years, he used alternative care methods such as meditation and vibrational healing within his endocrinology practice to help patients realize their ability to regenerate. In his book *Quantum Healing,* he describes how 98 percent of atoms that make up the human body will not be there one year from now. That is because every system in our body is built to respond to the stressful demands of life and regenerate to form an adapted, upgraded product. For example, when someone starts running on cement, they introduce increased forces to their bones, which signals the body to lay down stronger reinforcements (Wolff's law). That signal coordinates with osteoblasts and osteoclasts, which are small cells inside of bone that work to remodel the skeletal structure each day. This process eventually produces an entire new skeleton every three months in a healthy aging individual.[1] That fascinating healing schedule belongs solely to one of the eleven organ systems of the body, the skeletal system. The skin renews its layers each month, the lining of the stomach regenerates every four days, and the cells of the liver revamp the entire organ in six weeks. This endless operation of busy cell death and rebirth happens underneath our awareness as the surface brain focuses on higher-functioning activities. Even as a chiropractor, occasionally I will stop what I am methodically doing during a visit to stare at my healing hands. They are amazing! The skin of the hands creates a barrier toward pathogens and harsh chemicals, yet it maintains a vulnerability that allows me to feel tiny changes along the patient's body.

The intelligence packed into each microscopic building block of our being is almost overwhelming to comprehend. Just imagine how much there is to look at now in our environment. These brief and ethereal glimpses at our immediate world are a beautiful reminder to keep life in perspective. We are so magnificent yet wildly small and inconsequential to the overall flow of the universe. Each tiny being, combined with the health of those around us, will eventually form something big enough to have an impact on the planet—one in which healers are working to ensure it has a positive influence. Quantum medicine is the reminder I need to seamlessly look between the microscope of a medical imbalance and the telescope of a philosophical possibility. It asks providers to think of big-picture concepts that will influence subatomic particles to spark healing within the human spectrum of measurements. Part of this big-picture thinking leads a quantum healing supporter to address how invisible sources of electromagnetic waves can influence the energetic fields of a patient.

Making Waves

By viewing the body under the fine-tuned lens of quantum physics, you gain an appreciation for how balanced each cellular unit is within its own magnetic field. The body coordinates all its systems in response to numerous forms of intra/intercellular categories of communication while being monitored by fields of governing energy. Each cell in a healthy system of the body must communicate with coworkers in their local environment and report to different levels of management before reaching the big boss, the brain. The response from the brain follows descending pathways to deliver an action. Each level of management is a vital piece of the puzzle, one that your provider tries to reroute and restore during alternative health-care treatments.

I believe that the cellular communication of interest for quantum healing research is the influence that biophysical pressure waves have on living tissue. Cell receptors throughout the entire body are designed to receive information from mechanical stimulation to alert the body of detected changes in temperature, movement, tension, and incoming pressure waves. What is a pressure wave? Have you ever stood too close to the stage at a concert and felt like music coming from the stereo was pushing on your chest? The easiest pressure wave to relate to is the experience of a soundwave. While traveling through a medium such as air, a sound wave reaches the intricate acoustic system of our ear. The external ear receives a soundwave before passing the frequency through the middle ear's strategically placed eardrum and bones. As vibrations enter the fluid channels of the inner ear, coiling structures dampen the pressure and trigger the brain's response to changes in sound or equilibrium. This unique system is specifically built to accommodate pressure waves, but it is only one example of how those waves interfere and combine with our molecular function. This category of cellular communication suggests that different levels of energetic frequencies can influence our behavioral responses and health, all without our knowledge.

Invisible Intruders

Quantum physics teaches that there are resonant frequencies in the nucleus of each cell that are influenced by a constantly oscillating magnetic field.[7] Knowing this, we are led to question how easily the nucleus can be altered by invasive energies of vibrating waves and how quickly it snaps back to normal function once the waves are no longer present. Electromagnetic radiation is the result of combining electric fields with magnetic fields and can be measured along the light spectrum of EMF. Electromagnetic waves are classified according to wavelengths and frequency on the spectrum in image 7. It depicts the types of electromagnetic radiation within our universe.

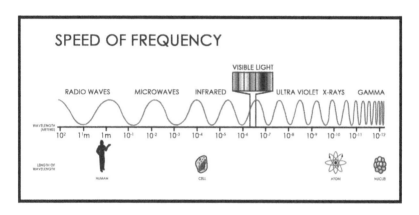

The higher the frequency (further to the right of image 7), the more energy is available to alter the chemical bonds between living cells. High ionizing frequencies of x-rays, for example, can produce harmful levels of radiation in comparison to low-frequency radio waves that hit the body without interfering with its chemistry (nonionizing). When chemical bonds are inappropriately severed by ionizing frequencies, unstable molecules are formed, known as free radicals. Electromagnetic waves that stimulate an increase in free radicals' level can disturb homeostasis systems such as the cardiovascular and nervous systems.[8]

I remember being a wide-eyed intern at my first job while the doctor demonstrated the effects that a cell phone had on a susceptible muscle unit in my body. First, he graded the muscle strength of my psoas major (a hip flexor) without the presence of my phone. Next, he asked me to hold my phone near a nerve plexus close to my heart or gut. While holding the phone to my chest, he retested my muscle strength. My helpless leg dropped as he effortlessly pressed it down toward the table. I laughed as I witnessed for the first time how an external electrical device could compete with my internal electricity. Following a treatment of chiropractic adjustments and some mentality work aimed at improving the emotional stimulus that the phone had on me, the same muscle test proved strong with or without my phone nearby. I don't enjoy using health care to entertain, so although I do not demonstrate examples of EMF influence in my daily care, I do try to offer my patients lifestyle behaviors to improve their daily interactions. Of all the protocols I use to treat people, questioning their interactions with electricity is not near the top of my list, but it has served a valuable purpose in cases that I struggled to resolve. An awareness of how technology influences your health is a rising necessity in our modern health-care regime. Lifestyle questions to consider when analyzing your daily EMF health include the following:

- Do you sit next to large electrical equipment at work each day?
- Is the electricity in your home updated and to code?
- How close do you sleep near electrical outlets and your cell phone?
- Do you wear a smartwatch every day and night?
- How many hours do you spend on a cell phone or with a laptop on your lap?
- Do you live close to an electric substation?

As a clinician, I aim to improve the awareness of existing interactions with invisible frequencies but in a realistic way—not as a scare tactic. Completely avoiding EMF is impossible, so realistically, we can decrease unnecessary exposure and maintain a resilient, healthy nervous system. Like the immune system combats the inevitable exposure to pathogens, a properly regulated electrical system allows the body to interact with moderate EMF without being negatively altered.

I could have been satisfied with the positive results that my patients were achieving by altering their EMF exposure, but I wanted to better understand the implications of how the brain, specifically the emotional brain, is influenced by EMF and radiation. Earlier in chapter 2, "Emotional Pain," I introduced the role that the hippocampus plays in the limbic system and converting recent memory to long-term memory. In a 2016 study, the scientists of Tabriz University watched as the hippocampus of their lab rats who were exposed to EMF fields for ten weeks became impaired. The results of that ten-week exposure, when exponentially applied to the decades of EMF influence that humans deal with, suggests alarming consequences. A healthy hippocampus is just one of the vital players in emotional regulation, behavioral motivation, and perception of healing capabilities. The review of their literature reports that neurological disorders caused by electromagnetic waves can result in surface symptoms such as memory loss, sleep disorders, headaches, and depression.[9]

The Conscious Connection with Vibrations

As I write this section of the book, my car sits lifelessly out front in the driveway with a dead battery. It is such an inconvenience within our easy world to lose the one generator that supports the entire function of a car. Accessible transportation has always comforted me. It offers the same sensation of freedom that the empowering ability of physical movement creates. Healthy movement is indicative of a healthy brain. If the generator of our body's power comes from the nervous system, is it operating at full capacity when the vehicle is struggling or drained of resources? A few authors and researchers have tried to quantify the vibrational amount of energy that a person is generating during different levels of emotional states. One of those authors, Dr. Joe Dispenza, describes in his research that as the frequency of matter increases, it will eventually "dematerialize" into orderly energy.[7] His work suggests that when a healthy, happily functioning person operates at this heightened level of electric frequency, the matter within our cellular structures vibrates so efficiently that energy transfer becomes "orderly" and optimally utilized. Highly functioning energy regulation allows for easy intake, utilization, and output of all of life's fueled actions.

Another author who dedicated his life to measuring the vibrational influence of emotional states is David Hawkins. The "Map of Consciousness" was introduced in his book *Power vs. Force* in 2014. On a scale, leveled from 0 to 1,000, his work demonstrates how emotions calibrate among the levels of ascending vibrations, correlating with the levels of a consciously aware person. In his eyes, that would be a person who is consciously aware of their role within the tangible world as well as their profound influence on the invisible world. As that peaceful and observant person emits a strong frequency, they will register high on the scale, far beyond someone who suffers from constant fear, guilt, and shame. His book goes into detail about the behavioral limitations of each stage and how famed figures of enlightenment would rank along the scale (Jesus Christ hit the ceiling at 1,000 with Gandhi close behind.) As I read, I wondered if the scale of consciousness could explain why some emotions were considered higher vibrationally than others, and, if so, how levels of energy could then influence the chemistry of the body.

I was taught to abide by Hawkins's Map of Consciousness from healing mentors who believed that healthy internal dialogue created healing. "If you want to practice energy work, you'll need to advance to a higher level of consciousness and self-awareness." So, I learned the system, its implication of how my emotions could affect my health, and then tried to align my life with David's impression of ascending consciousness. While these topics were successful in helping patients find relief from pain, I struggled personally to feel like I was progressing on my own ascension journey. I lived out of fear that I would register low on the scale and for a time, lost sight of my initial mission to heal alongside my patients or yoga students. If I was asking my community to trust their ability to heal, there was no room for doubting my own innate gifts.

In my current practice, I have stepped away from this grading scale, but I do recommend the book to intuitive healers and anyone who enjoys an intriguing read. I now choose to endorse any level of consciousness that encourages us to become aware of the thoughts we naturally engage with and how those thoughts can dictate our pain, emotions, and behavior. Our thoughts are easily influenced by interpersonal interactions and media, so be wary of the resilience we acquire from consistent stimuli of violent television and argumentative social media posts. It takes practice to learn how to witness experiences in a detached way; to be able to view how triggers affect your mood and physical responses. Mindfulness practices that help with improving this self-awareness will be discussed further in the next two chapters, "Yoga Philosophy" and "Mental Dialogue."

What Is a Medical Intuitive?

> I felt a great disturbance in the force.
> — Obi-Wan Kenobi

As my practice deepened, I grew used to laughing with patients after restoring muscles that were comically weak moments before to full force. Their limited joint range of motion melted away for the first time in six years in just one thirty-minute session. I didn't know how to explain why I was drawn to mobilizing their ankles to improve neck flexion, but they trusted me, which forced me to trust myself. The ability to communicate with a subconscious portion of living things comes down to trust. The longer my clinical, skeptically trained brain battled to make sense of how science would explain these experiences, the longer it took my patients to get better. I would later learn that the gut instincts I was experiencing are called medical intuition.

Caroline Myss is a renowned medical intuitive and spiritual healer who laughs at the number of her workshop attendees that are disappointed to discover that she believes intuition and symbolic sight are not a gift but a trained skill. She considers intuition to be a trainable ability to listen to the instinctual messages of your body and to then make decisions in alignment with that urge. "Intuition is neither the ability to engage prophesy nor a means of avoiding loss or pain. It is the ability to use energy data to make decisions in the immediate moment. Energy data are the emotional, psychological, and spiritual components of a given situation. They are the 'here and now' ingredients of life, not nonphysical information from some future place or guide."

The Benefits of Intuitive (Quantum) Medicine

While writing this book, I had to remember that many of the people reading it will not have an existing alternative health-care routine. Why would they feel called to start implementing something that doesn't seem relevant or necessary? So, for those wondering, "why is an intuitive care provider—a medical professional who believes in the collective health of your tangible and intangible body—a necessity to seek out?" In the simplest of terms, I would say that everyone should have a doctor on their round table of healers who is not afraid to ask, "Why?" When patients that I cotreat come into my office with referrals for surgery or a new medicine, I respectfully ask, "Did you ask why your doctor prescribed that before a trial period of noninvasive care or dietary alterations?" I don't want to shoot the messenger (the patient in between numerous modalities of health care), but I do want each patient to take responsibility for their own health trajectory; to know what options there are. Under the heat of a confident doctor, can you look them in the eye to ask, "Why am I receiving this injection today?" or "Is this medicine absolutely necessary?" And "If it is, what are the potential side effects and time frame that we'll trial being on it?"

Medical providers who believe in the electromagnetic balance that governs the body tend to be minimalists, in any field. An MD who leans toward the natural aspect of a DO may recommend fewer checkups or prescription medicine to encourage patients to view their own symptoms as less severe and personally manageable. In chiropractic school, I was taught to assume that if I refer a patient to an orthopedic surgeon for anything, that they would most likely receive a surgery; "if the only tool you have as a doctor is a hammer, then everything will look like a nail." This outdated argument assumes that surgeons perform surgery just like massage therapists supply massages— on everyone they service. I believe the trend of our integrative health system is leaning toward an autonomous process where doctors of unique specialties now sacrifice income to refer patients to the proper caretaker. I like to believe that I can offer anyone who walks in my door some type of pain relief or comfort, but that does not mean they are each a candidate for chiropractic care or musculoskeletal rewiring.

Finding a health-care provider who delves into both the subconscious mind and the electromagnetic body will sooner recognize the body's needs than someone who doesn't know to look. At some point along each of our healing journeys, we will find a provider, a hobby, or a mentor that will strengthen our ability to choose the thoughts we engage with and compel us to observe the interactions of our world in a new light.

Counterarguments and Taking Precautions

If you've found alternative care during a time of struggling health or self-doubt, be careful not to be too eager when grabbing for advice from someone you hold in high regard. Physical and emotional stress can cloud the instinctive judgment of a patient as well as the provider you entrust. While working and utilizing the services of healers who study energy medicine, I have come across desperate patients who, while crying, ask me to give personal life advice based on my intuition. That is both inconsiderate and outside my professional skill set to provide any answer beyond a referral to the appropriate counselor. It is difficult to create firm boundaries while showing empathy for a patient, but for degree holders, there is a fine line between sympathetic conversation and medical advice. I have been mentored by numerous yoga therapists and energy providers who have lost track of their medical reality. Like all enlightenment journeys, we are here to have a human experience and must maintain a healthy life balance on the horizontal plane, no matter how fun or enticing the vertical plane may seem.

Lacking balance and a safe learning pace feels like burning the candle from both ends. Clinically, I went off the deep end in 2019 and briefly lost track of my original foundations in medicine. I am grateful to have experienced the extremes of meditation and yogic sensations because the detachment from reality that I experienced enabled me to witness gifts that I would never have believed from a secondhand story. While disconnected living can be easier than facing life's challenges, I am very thankful for the supportive people in my life who quietly observed my transition but then pulled me back to earth when it was the right time. Not everyone that I took this philosophical journey with was able to come back to a safe mindset before crossing a professional boundary. Fortunately, I kept a level head during the time of self-inquiry and made most of my private areas of study exactly that—private.

Energetic Education

To a layperson, perfectly common and accepted medical procedures can seem like magic at times. It is the responsibility of a provider to properly present the difference between procedures taught in their credentialing curriculum and auxiliary practices that were acquired during personal study. I never miss the chance during treatment to explain to a patient when we've transferred from chiropractic medicine to an alternative method. I want them to know the difference, especially if they have never been to a chiropractor before. I tell them, "I am a unique first experience!" Extracurricular techniques studied outside of endorsed teaching institutions often reward an attendee with a certificate of completion, but this weekend training does not indicate medical training nor should it derail the direction of a medical care plan. Under the guidance of someone with skewed motives or a large ego, influential patients can get taken advantage of during the ascending process. Using safe communication styles and respecting professional boundaries, we as healers can prevent these students from avoiding natural medicine in the future.

Energetic bodywork and intuitive medicine are growing fields within our society, but their influence is being slowed down due to an inability to reproduce objective results for studying purposes. Most patients, in any realm of healthcare, are not aware of current research and supported evidence, so they place their trust in the provider of their choosing and develop an understanding for medical interventions based on the progress they receive. Due to a high prevalence of misunderstood bodywork, the reputation of alternative techniques suffers and contributes to the limited support necessary for further learning and safe application. When abiding by the law and clearly identifying the line between a hunch and a medical diagnosis, what can it hurt if someone claims they are a medical intuitive? I remind myself of this when I witness people who abuse their power of influence; it is not the superhuman gifts that are the problem. It is the human weaknesses that tarnish the reputation of a growing field and limit the beneficial impact that the information could have on a patient.

So how should someone navigate safely while blending health care and intuition? The answer is simple — step by step. I present the information of this book in a sequence of chapters that I know will safely deliver anyone interested in higher levels of healing to a safe destination, for both a practice and a personal lifestyle. For providers who get an instinctive hunch while treating with your foundational skill set, listen to it but address it in a medically sound way. For example, while I was recently treating a man for low back pain after working a long shift at a mechanic shop, a brief image of an anatomical kidney flashed through my mind. The inappropriate way to communicate my gut instinct would be to say, "I'm seeing that you are suffering from kidney dysfunction." This implies a diagnosis without any medical testing or legal justification for creating a treatment plan aimed at improving his kidney. The appropriate way to address an intuitive hunch would be to blend clinical prompt questions into the treatment conversation, such as, "I'd like to rule out any internal referral mechanisms for your back pain. Have you suffered from any urinary cramping or signs of infection?" Depending on how much you trust your instincts, you may let their denial of symptoms close the conversation.

For this gentleman, I knew he was not very body conscious and needed to experience high levels of pain before mentally becoming aware of a health imbalance. I completed my care that day with a referral to see his primary care physician to rule out kidney issues. I sent him a prescription for a urinalysis and lumbar spine x-rays, due to low back pain that was not responding to conservative care. The next week, my patient returned to my office and reported that he was suffering from kidney stones! Would a less intuitive provider have gotten to the same conclusion? Probably, but maybe not as fast or before intense pain surfaced. It is truly semantics; health-care professionals are taught to recognize visceral signs of disruption on the surface and may call a situation like this a differential diagnosis, but for someone who believes in their ability to safely apply intuition into a medical practice, I call it both.

Practice Feeling Energy

If intrigued by the concept of energy medicine and emotional pain, you may be wondering where to find examples of energy transfer at home. I recommend that you start by recalling the difference between a high-energy day and a low-energy day. What we write off as low blood sugar levels or sleep deprivation may have an extra component of electrical imbalance. For patients who are struggling to dissipate the stressors of life throughout their physical body, I remind them to view energy as fuel for physical exertion and to find a creative outlet to burn some electricity off! I'll explain.

If energy cannot be created or destroyed, then in theory, it is passed between living creatures and should transmute into the form of energy needed to create movement, heat, and life reactions. I believe that creative outlets offer a venue to burn off excess energy that either doesn't belong to you or no longer serves the energy requirements of your ascending self. I prefer orchestrated and detoxifying movements like yoga or running, but not all creation involves exercise. Dancing, singing, painting, or playing a musical instrument are all forms of energetic output that require us to be focused and present with our feelings. With the right intention, I dedicate certain activities to "using unhealthy or foreign energy in my body to fuel my healing session." I always feel better afterward and make a mental note to transform the negativity that left me into a higher and purer source of energy that someone else can benefit from.

One of the easiest ways to introduce invisible force is to feel an energy with your own hands. Start by rubbing your hands together until heat builds between them. Very slowly, begin to pull the hands apart and notice the increased sensations you've created. By generating thermal energy from friction, the receptors in our skin can easily recognize heat and temperature changes. Eventually, as the distance between the hands grows too large, the energy created diffuses back into the external environment and is no longer detectable as "hot" or "present." Try this rubbing exercise again. Even slower than the first time, pull your hands apart one centimeter. Toy with subtle movements of each finger and each palm to detect small signs of invisible pressure, magnetism, or resistance emitted from the space between the hands.

Some students report recognizing a pulling force that keeps the hands from separating farther until they overpower the magnetism and open past its barrier. Others are drawn to the resistant forces that feel as if there is an object inside the palms that pushes back when closing the distance between the two hands. Over time, practicing this awareness will aid in healing techniques for yourself or on another person. Like developing the palpation skills needed for chiropractic sciences, practice is the only way to improve the neurological feedback in the hands. As sensitivity to changes in energy improves, you will be able to feel signs of heat, pressure, or magnetism at wide distances between the hands. This skill will be a vital component for someone who is interested in learning techniques such as acupuncture or chakra healing. Chakras are the energy centers of the yogic *subtle body* and will be thoroughly discussed in the following chapter on yoga philosophy.

Review Questions and Focus Points

I am not the first to explain the complex aspects of quantum healing nor the most qualified translator, but I will happily aid its popularity and growth. By opening our minds to its existence and looking for opportunities for it to relate to daily life, we accelerate society's journey toward the scientific and medical advances necessary to harness the power of a quantum reality. One step at a time! The takeaways from this chapter are listed below.

1. Stay observant of your daily movements and physical sensations beyond tired, hungry, and stressed. See the small signs of life that we robotically pass each day.

2. Maintain an awareness of your body's reaction and interaction with other people, plants, and technology. Does the pain or anxiety you're experiencing belong to you?

3. Identify which life triggers are categorized as low vibrational and harmful.

4. Maintain efforts to surround yourself with high and healthy vibrational experiences.

5. View your life circumstances and physical sensations as temporary; remember how fluid and adaptable the body is. Even if it is slow, change is always there. Help your body and mind along each step of change to slowly build each phase higher toward ascension.

Review Questions

1. Have you ever walked out of a doctor's office feeling offended that they didn't give you the medicine you expected or the attention you felt your symptoms warranted?

2. Based on their recommendations, assign who played the role of healer. (Options can include: You, the doctor, a medicine, or an intervention)

3. Did that provider place blame for your health issues or leave you with the open-ended sense that things could improve?

4. Revisit questions one 1 through 3 but using the example of a doctor you hold in high regard. How do the answers vary from the first time you went through the process?

   Use this exercise to identify if you have an internal or external locus of control, meaning you believe that someone else is in control of your health or, ultimately, that you are.

5. What types of physical/mental/emotional/spiritual ailments do you categorize under those two perceptions? (For example, "I know that my sporadic low back pain, stomach cramps, and anxious tendencies are in my control, but if I have chest tightness, I'm calling the doctor immediately.")

6. Try listening to a recording of Tibetan singing bowls or a gong bath and journal on your body's response.

In yoga, there is a belief that the mind
is more powerful than matter.
Where do you think the saying came from?
— David R. Hawkins, *Power vs. Force*

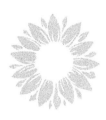

CHAPTER 6

Yoga Philosophy

Why I First Stepped onto a Mat

Like many others, I broke the yoga ice while seeking an exercise that I could do quickly at home or in the back of my office over lunch without sweating too much. To avoid public shame, I stayed in the comfort of my own home for over a year while practicing. On YouTube, I watched "real yogis" like Sadie Nardini to challenge my athletic body until I felt confident enough to take my practice to a public studio. I hid in the back, judging each person as harshly as I did my own body. As a previous athlete, I didn't like to witness my own limitations, and the poses within yoga easily showcased every muscle, joint, and limb that I had neglected or incorrectly trained for the previous decade. I'd never guess it at the time, but that unattractive and uncomfortable yoga practice was shaping much more than my physique.

Healing Insight—Yoga

The *asanas* of yoga (pronounced ah-sah-nahs) are the physical poses that the body can create during this organized movement practice. The poses are representations of the beautiful things in our universe, such as mountains, dolphins, or my favorite flower, a bird of paradise. By using the structure of the body to symbolically morph into these creations, we unlock new skills and perspectives that help us live a better life. There are considered eight categories within yoga's philosophy, and while the physical poses only make up one of the eight "limbs," they are the most recognized depiction of yoga in our Western culture. I am an advocate for teaching students and patients the physical portion of yoga because I believe it is a wonderful place to begin a journey inward. Most often, this beneficial practice of stretching, breathing, and thinking will naturally develop toward the other limbs of yoga's teachings. Yoga—at its purest form—can be anything you need it to be. I joke that on a scale between a hamstring stretch and a spiritual awakening, yoga is anything you make of it. I now incorporate much more than tight muscles or properly placed bones into my yoga experience, but the asanas are what first caught my attention and converted me into a lifelong enthusiast.

During a yoga class, an instructor will verbally guide students through a template of poses called a sequence, calling out things like "Sun salutation A or B." Each sequence will match the unique training of the teacher or studio's values. There are many different styles of yoga, all stemming from historic innovators and their lineages of teachings. Names like Krishnamacharya, BKS Iyengar, Pattabhi Jois, and Baron Baptiste have all inspired a specific branch of philosophy that has left a permanent imprint on the yoga community. In this brief introduction to yoga philosophy and its demographics, I hope to ignite an interest that propels your personal healing journey. I will address a few of the limbs of yoga and why I believe everyone has access to creating a self-sustaining yoga routine in their daily life.

Getting Started

For most, entering a yoga class for the first time is very intimidating, so before pulling the trigger, determine how much accountability you'll need to maintain a sustainable practice. I think having an accountability partner (a.k.a. a friend) to meet at yoga makes the first experience more accessible and it encourages you to enjoy the community in addition to any physical benefits. With a safety network on the mat next to you, try numerous styles of yoga and at different times of the day. Similarly to chiropractic, finding the technique that matches the specific stage of your journey will only come with trial experiments. Flow through the uncharted territory and trust that if your body responds positively, then you have found your current movement medicine.

Many students practice yoga at home, which saves money, needing to find a babysitter, and travel time. If you choose to become a stay-at-home practitioner, I encourage you to create a quiet area dedicated to yoga so that each time you step onto the mat, all attention goes to personal progress and avoids distraction. At some point, I hope you branch out and take your developing practice into a studio. The benefits of utilizing a studio include the guided safety cues in poses, variation of sequences, accountability to practice, and community involvement. We learn best by mirroring others, so when exposed to a group of students, you will progress faster.

If you have physical limitations and are concerned how your body will respond to yoga, I highly recommend private yoga sessions. Private one-on-one classes are perfect for beginners who feel overwhelmed in typical class settings. Sessions are designed to create safe and specific sequences for your body type, capability, and previous injuries. There is no better way to personally improve flexibility, balance, and strength.

What's Your In-Between?

Throughout my athletic and clinical experience, I've witnessed training trends come and go, taking the damaging effects with them. I cringe when high school or young college athletes suffer from debilitating back pain as if they had the spine of someone twice their age. I believe the prevalence of early spinal injuries stems from the imbalance between hours spent as a sedentary student and an active mover. The harder we learn and work, the more our lifestyle is confined to a chair. Typically, to make up for sitting, we go to the gym after work for a few hours of high-intensity training without any casual activity between extremes.

In chiropractic school, yoga became my in-between activity. It satisfied the urge to move without making myself more exhausted. Eventually, the practice became my warmup, the meat of the routine, and my cooldown, depending on what I needed that day. This was the freedom I was looking for in an exercise outlet—to help my mental health match how good I felt on the outside. It was drastically different from the resilient, hardened mentality that most competitive sports required, as if a high pain tolerance is a bragging right.

I spent years finding myself deep within the poses of yoga, hopping between studios, workshops, and yoga buddies. Eventually, this hopping taught me a lot about my preferences within the vast range of yoga styles, teachers, and beliefs. I loved the powerful athletic flows that kept me in shape. The never-ending sequences of stretching, breathing, and strengthening perfectly complemented other forms of exercise that I already loved, such as running and rock climbing. Those classes were a great way to connect with other healthy women, but even as I learned inversions or fancy arm-balancing postures, I still had a firm opinion on how far my progress could reach.

It took a grueling ankle fracture from a women's indoor soccer game to slow down my athletic practice and make me analyze my "success" as a student of yoga. This heavy phase of healing introduced me to restorative yoga, which taught me an emotional resilience that power yoga didn't require or provide space for. While enduring the pain, I journeyed through personal false realities and their effect on the physical outcomes of my yoga poses. Before I could reap the benefits of any practice, I had to sit still, feel my pain, and thaw my frozen athletic mindset. As my ankle healed, I felt years of soccer melt away, releasing access to new spaces in which to breathe, move, and play. Each time I stepped onto a mat, my body seemed less obstinate and almost cooperative. Positions that were recently difficult became a familiar place to dock my mind and settle the emotions that stirred within. It is because of this freedom I found within my own physical temple that I wanted to dive into the depths of yoga and to become a teacher. I had to learn the benefits of each pinch, doubt, and fear in the poses before I could spread healing knowledge to others.

Opening My Heart through Yoga

> You will never reach your full potential
> if you don't open your heart.
> —Paulo Coelho

Not only was 2018 my first full year of practicing as a chiropractor, but it was also the year I decided to commit to a six-month teacher training program in Fayetteville, Arkansas. I spent most of my weekends taking yoga seminars and reading all the books I could find about yogic theories, anatomical explanations, and mechanical properties of the yoga poses. I did a lot of research to identify why yoga was gaining popularity so I could help more people find the practice. I was looking for a competitive edge in the chiropractic realm and I wanted to offer a safe transition into yoga for people who would not have found it otherwise. What originally began as a plan to earn more chiropractic patients, turned into a beautiful opportunity to create more yoga students. As a chiropractor, I fell in love with the mechanical flow of bodies in motion and I now had a way to combine the two worlds in my life!

My personal yoga practice was accelerated by becoming a private yoga instructor, registered yoga teacher, and an instructor for yoga teacher training. These roles helped me to blend chiropractic, rehabilitative sciences, and specialized yoga training into a package that I could deliver wholeheartedly to those who were also eager to heal. Yoga's addition into my chiropractic care gave patients something to look forward to after resolving injuries. The heightened control that they gained through adjustments and neurological rewiring was beautifully showcased through yoga postures before advancing to higher level concepts such as self-inquiry and self-exploration. These teachings were a natural complement to the emotional healing techniques I was offering. It encouraged patients to address imbalances at home and to invite their families to grow alongside of their improvements.

Your Vibe Attracts Your Tribe

It is human nature to crave
intimacy and belonging,
which is essential preventative medicine.
Copious scientific data proves
that loneliness is a greater
risk to your health than smoking
or lack of exercise. Finding
your tribe is better than any vitamin,
diet, or exercise regimen.
— Lisa Rankin, *The Health Benefits of Finding Your Tribe*

Not only do yoga practitioners love to feel good; they also love to connect with like-minded people and become advocates for community platforms that have enriched their lives. Personal contact and emotional support play a large role in our ability to cope with life stressors, influencing how we individually experience levels of physical pain. The familiarity of kind faces at a local yoga studio attracts those who are lacking a supportive network. Routine exposure to a healthy group of individuals is the perfect medicine for anyone needing to feel accepted or at home within themselves.

As a doctor, yoga instructor, and studio-hopping student, I love the support networks that yoga studios have evolved into. What was once home to solely physical support, is now a home for social and educational resources as well. You don't need to be a medical student to receive quality health information anymore. The comfort of learning new or intimidating material in a familiar space offers members affordable access to highly intelligent and qualified people. Workshops, seminars, and certification programs fill the schedules of successful yoga studios. Modern studios now assume the role of a community center; what were once considered businesses for yoga are now home to recovery programs, hands-on manual therapy, mental health discussions, spiritual gatherings, nutritional planning, and wellness festivals. Studios often host celebrity guest speakers and employ weekly instructors who hold other professional, medical credentials.

I love that yoga students have a place to go where they feel safe enough to ask about musculoskeletal concerns and self-healing options. Medical providers only have exposure to a limited population of patients who can afford care or will rely on insurance coverage to start their healing. To fill in the gaps, I have to trust that the recommendations of certified yoga instructors will care for the musculoskeletal community that I will never meet. They are frontline wellness providers! Yoga teachers have a foundational knowledge of the human structure that allows them to offer postural advice, modifications for exercise, and breathing cues that can restore a misaligned nervous system. Working on those three areas, in my experience, can resolve most aches and pains. I also truly respect when an instructor recognizes that a student's pain is beyond the aid of yogic training and that a medical referral is necessary. Within these classes, I have found that the title of a yoga teacher or a chiropractor truly represents a collection of jobs, such as a movement coach, a translator, and an intuitive healer.

Awareness of Self

> We do not learn from experience …
> we learn from reflecting on experience.
> — John Dewey

One of the most beneficial practices of yoga studies is the section called *svadhyaya*, or simply put, self-inquiry. The practice of self-reflection and self-study is a beautiful introduction to witnessing your own unraveling, and I can attest to its effective healing of the mind, the body, and the spirit. For many, yoga is the first outlet where approachable healers ask you to sit down, witness the emotions and behaviors that constitute your reality, and then share them with strangers.

Historically, this is not the section of a yoga practice that lures in a young crowd, but the rapidly changing popularity of yoga now includes more intellectual branches. Because yoga studios ideally represent a setting that cultivates the image of non-judgment, progress, and enlightenment, many students feel safe to vulnerably unravel their challenges here. High school and college students are resorting to yoga communities to learn how to adapt to stressful lifestyles and, by doing so, stumble upon a greater sense of self-awareness. I find that yoga is a daily menu for your soul. Do you want to order a sweat and a stretch for your hamstrings? Perfect, we have classes for that! If instead you are looking for answers about your energetic body and its connection to the universe, we have that too. A physical yoga practice will open the door for you to cultivate awareness of mental self-talk, physical resistances, and your healing abilities. When we begin practicing yoga with the intention to heal and connect on a deeper level, something magical and beyond logic starts to happen.

As explained in *The Four Agreements,* "Awareness is always the first step because if you are not aware, there is nothing you can change." When you are ready, a yoga practice will naturally bring you closer to an internal unknown. In a yogic world, the energetic being that emanates from within our physical boundaries is called a *subtle body.* The subtle body is described as a deep existence that offers subtle signs of intelligent life on the tangible surface. This energetically vibrating part of our human experience, once felt, opens the bigger doors needed to trust in spirituality.

Craving Something Bigger Than Us

Yoga certainly isn't the only group gathering that serves to utilize the strength of a collective to achieve better versions of ourselves. Self-inquiry is often encouraged by spiritual and physical practices like yoga or religious groups, and it can help us to process limiting emotions that fuel a sense of isolation. With less walls and more clarity, we learn to communicate with the subtle body. For those who are resistant to the practice of yoga, please recognize that students drawn to the community created in yoga studios are benefiting from the same love and comfort that you may find in church worship, support groups, and therapy sessions. Each of these gathering styles provides faith with an outlet to bloom.

I believe that yoga is such a powerful practice because in addition to a spiritual sense of connection, students have an attention focusing routine to better understand sensations, alter unpleasantries, and witness the immediate benefits of mindful movement. Yoga, like all mindful movement, doesn't ask an anxious mind to focus on the unknown future. The practice asks you to have faith that the present efforts you are demonstrating will lead you somewhere forward and up. Students learn to trust each step because they can feel the tiny signs of progress, even if there are no obvious signs on the surface. You can watch someone practice yoga or read about it for years, but you can't begin to embody a deep knowing of your subtle body until you have a personal experience. As you do, you'll begin to see intuition as I do—an innate gift and prerequisite for true healing.

While most people go to yoga to improve their physical needs, those who stick with it gain a whole new outlook on life. Yoga can be a place to finally experience the connection between the power of our mind and its ability to alter the physical world. Many have heard of the term *consciousness* and probably affiliate it with new age vocabulary. Consciousness is defined as the state of being aware of something, either within or surrounding yourself. Traditionally, yoga participants are considered highly conscious people who have an eye for bigger-picture ideas and can easily see the world beyond their personal concerns.

Yoga students are extremely concerned about their health, the environment, and the community, so most practitioners are also conservationists. This is the reason that most sustainable companies and eco-friendly ventures are affiliated with yogis, hippies, and environmentalists. Can you truly support love and healing without wanting those things for the lives around you as well? When you put highly conscious people together, changes are bound to happen—cumulative and exponential changes for those involved and for the people they are in contact with in the community.

Empathetic Listening

Yoga classes offer an environment to intimately sit next to and witness other people who are going through the same problems. I love sitting in a class and scanning the room beforehand to gauge what my students are there for. Their bodies cannot hide the internal stress, relationship struggles, surgeries, fear, or seclusion that they harbor, so I aim to talk in generalized prompts during a class to help each student release their own resistances to emotional healing.

Throughout this guide, I anticipate that readers will question why I think it is within my right and scope of practice to discuss emotions and mentality with patients. I am a chiropractor, not a talk therapist after all. Please understand that this overlap happens within every medical field; patients build a relationship with providers and continue to unravel layers of need until that specialized doctor transfers the job responsibility with appropriate referrals. I view the gray area of scope of practice like this: If I am a trusted and familiar outlet for a patient to disclose potentially harmful emotions, I respect that responsibility and allow them to share. Cutting off a patient's cry for help due to practice limitations feels inhumane and may discourage the person from ever bringing it up again (in any medical office). Most health-care providers are trained to recognize red flags that dictate immediate referrals, but it takes a lot of experience to formulate approachable communication styles that create space for this.

The emotional dialect that I use in practice truly stemmed from yoga teacher training. I've taken numerous psychology courses in my years of college and postgraduate studies, all of which were taught to pass tests and recognize when it was appropriate to refer someone to a therapist. Yoga training was the first curriculum that encouraged me to talk to people like a human, not their doctor. Yoga philosophy created a safe space that demonstrated that healing—a fundamental human right—was our highest obligation to share with humankind. Without a license, without liability protection, without a protocol to follow for insurance, the self-inquiry section of yoga teacher training encouraged each of us to truly look at another person, empathetically listen, and freely respond as an equal person. It was a liberating process— learning to analyze and respond to a human from a perspective that wasn't trying to diagnose an issue or nip the story due to time constraints. And to learn this from women who had no formal medical education? I was in awe of how experienced the yoga leaders were in areas that I lacked. This stage of training would profoundly enhance my ability to connect with and truly hear the subliminal messages from my patients thereafter.

To improve your interpersonal communication, research helpful topics such as trauma-informed yoga certifications and empathetic listening. Then go practice your new skills with yoga groups or with public-speaking companies like Toastmasters International.

Meditation Medicine

> You are the universe experiencing itself.
> — Alan Watts, *Become What You Are*

I have found that yoga is a personal lesson on mindful movement that reminds you of your ability to alter life. While focusing on personal interests such as decreasing pain and fear of injury, you learn that the shape of life has shaped your body. What seems like a simple stretch or trying to balance on one leg can open your eyes to how distracted life has become. Luckily, the same magic works in reverse. You can shape your mind or body to reshape life. Yoga is an amazing bridge to connect the physical experience with the underlying subconscious challenges of being a human. That is why I describe yoga as an excavation process. If used daily, it offers each participant a chance to dig deeply into the mind-body and reveal how far from a normal and comfortable baseline we've come. Practicing throughout the week will also offer a glimpse into what stress has truly been placed on daily posture and compensatory systems.

After the excavation process, a yoga practice provides highly concentrated sensations to support both your mind and body through the next stage of self-development, which becomes meditation. As a new student learns to move, breathe, and rest in restorative yoga poses, they are almost tricked into trying meditation. Meditation now has many forms and styles, but this mysterious activity has been linked to peace, serenity, and improved health for decades. A few sessions per week provide calming and reassuring support that will promote healing and positive physiological effects.

The Stress Response

The chemical physiology of being stressed is the key to understanding why so many practitioners recommend meditating. All stressful triggers of life, whether we are conscious of their influence or not, initiate the sympathetic nervous system (SNS) via the fight-or-flight stress response. This response describes how stress causes a cascade of changes in the body that can be highly beneficial in the short term but drastically destructive over the long term. Some stress, called *eustress*, is good to motivate us to exercise or respond well to challenges. The constant feeling of being anxiously aroused (*distress*) is the concerning stimulation that will wear down your body's immune system and willpower simultaneously.

When stress rules the body, you are running on fight-or-flight mode. During this process, the body turns its back on maintaining the regulation and function of any system that doesn't provide priority survival instincts, such as digestion and sexual organs. Because of this, chronically stressed individuals will then experience disturbed hormonal cycles and gastric abnormalities until the nervous system can find sustainable ease to again offer essential energy to run secondary systems. Priorities for a human living in sympathetic survival mode include a high heart rate capacity, easy respiration, prepared brain power, and quick-responding muscular activation. While the priority systems are stealing the energy of a stressed body preparing to fight or flee, it is poorly equipped to restore and heal.

Cortisol's Role in Stress

Sitting above both kidneys, the adrenal glands produce vital chemicals, including cortisol, a steroid hormone. At normal levels, cortisol is responsible for controlling blood sugar, metabolism, and balancing blood pressure. While the sympathetic nervous system is in overdrive due to the stress response, the adrenal glands pump out excessive amounts of cortisol. When this steroid hormone is present in high levels, it will suppress the immune system and predispose the body to infection or disease.[1] The excess cortisol then depletes neurotransmitters, such as norepinephrine (alert), dopamine (snuggle), and serotonin (pleasure) from working correctly. Without these neurotransmitters in the brain, it is difficult to feel alert, experience pleasurable feelings, or maintain a positive mood. Negative emotions enhance pro-inflammatory cytokines (proteins secreted by the immune system) which in excess, cause inflammation and delay wound or injury healing.[2]

Within the limbic system of the brain (Refer to Image 2), stress causes excess levels of cortisol to be released, which wears down the brain centers that process and store emotional memories. This prevents the limbic system from forming new and healthy memories while the stress persists.[3] Limbic-cortical mappings of experience are maps grounded in the limbic system which generate the organization of consciousness (our interpretation and reaction to experience).[4] I'll further discuss how those interpretations can become distorted and blocked in the next chapter.

Making Waves

Dr. Lisa Rankin explains in her book *Mind Over Medicine*, "Some of my sickest patients are the ones drinking green organic shakes every day and running marathons. Their bodies are seemingly healthy, but their minds are sick." Diet, exercise, chiropractic, yoga, and sleep cover a fraction of the full spectrum of healing. Even with such a regimen, we can live in a state of stress. Chiropractors often see phantom symptoms that manifest from stress such as backaches, headaches, dizziness, fatigue, insomnia, and GI distress. Alternative modalities like acupuncture and yoga aim to release pent up emotions through mental focus to improve the symptoms that chemical stress has caused. The relaxation response from meditative practices plays a pivotal role in reversing the effects of the stress response.

When the mind is soothed, levels of cortisol decrease, allowing blood pressure and neurological components, such as neurotransmitters, to be restored. Dopamine, a goal-oriented hormone, improves the pleasure center in the brain. Oxytocin, the cuddle hormone, is responsible for decreasing inflammation while activating serotonin and stimulating the release of endorphins.[3] Serotonin lifts our mood and inhibits the hypersensitive amygdala. Meanwhile, endorphins, nature's natural morphine, trigger dopamine release to reduce pain and give you that runner's high feeling.

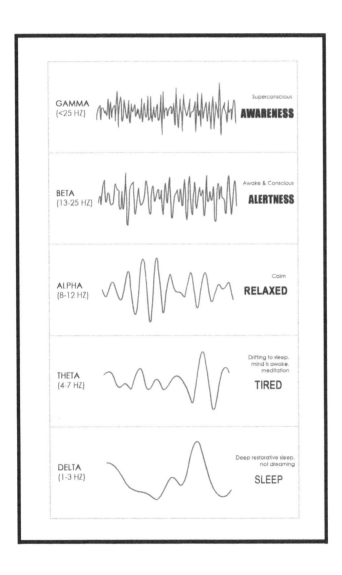

Through the process of meditating, stress levels and heart rates are reduced as you simultaneously alter the brain waves. When the body is aware and actively awake, the brain produces electric waves at a high frequency, known as beta waves. (See Image 8) During the rare period when the body and mind relax, brain wave frequencies become lower and are classified as alpha, theta, and delta waves.[3] Delta waves are predominantly experienced during a deep sleep. The more time and practice you dedicate to meditation, the easier it is to achieve those deeply relaxed brain waves without falling asleep. These slow brain waves promote healing because the relaxation response allows your body to rejuvenate and heal itself.

For everyday application, take this information to create a new interest and do your own research on meditation; some of us need a little more proof of the benefits before deciding to adopt a new habit. Remember that the goal of stress reduction with meditation is not to remove stressful triggers from your life. The goal is to help you become more aware of the invisible triggers and then more resilient to those stressful situations. Regular meditation encourages you to view life events with a level head, so instead of reacting to them, you are calm enough to choose your response. Staying on top of our responses to life in a conscious way maintains our health at a subconscious level.

I fell in love with meditation not because I learned stillness but because it allowed me to better appreciate movement. At the end of a yoga class or movement practice, the stark difference of not moving is an amazing reward. The surrendering of all efforts after a demanding effort helps the brain apply and integrate the recent movement patterns. Then at the end of meditation, you reintroduce tiny movements with an acute sense of awareness that increases the sensation in every finger or facial muscle. The surge of information to the brain helps you appreciate how much coordination and communication goes into larger movements. After seven years of practice, I still reap the benefits of that contrast; somewhere between meditation's stillness and yoga's movements, I find myself.

What Is the Point of Stretching?

There is this idea in some yoga circles
that we have to force ourselves into a pose.
Yoga must be modified to fit you,
not the other way around.
— Indra Devi

As a sports-minded doctor, I was drawn to the styles of yoga that showcased the intricacies of anatomy in motion. Everyone has a different degree of tissue flexibility and bony alignment based on their genetic build, developmental movement patterns, previous injuries, and present occupational positions. For some, yoga is a natural progression of an old activity like dancing or cheerleading, so they have a larger range of pain-free motion before reaching a stretch. For less active individuals or novices, the range of pain-free motion may be extremely tiny or nonexistent. It is more challenging to encourage this type of patient to commit to a trial of yoga, so instead of explaining the benefits of yoga alone, I focus on highlighting how yoga complements their favorite activity or mandatory daily movements.

That discussion brings us to the science within a stretch mechanism and the joint nourishment that movement provides. We are about to get technical so read in small spurts, take a break to practice the movement, and mark this page to come back to as a reference.

As you dedicate yourself to an organized stretching routine (like yoga), new thresholds of a stretch are created. The beginning of movement without a stretch is an easy, familiar range of motion that you barely notice. Walking, standing, rolling over in bed, or crossing your legs; your brain has completed these motions so many that it has a stored expectation of simplicity. Previously wired motor patterns coordinate the joints, muscles, and the balance necessary to return to the easy movement on command. Past this effortless zone is where a stretch begins, but before that gets uncomfortable, there is a brief period of simple resistance where the body notices it's nearing the end of an effortless range of motion. It's not alarmed yet, just alert.

Within every muscle belly is a stretch receptor known as a muscle spindle that detects changes in length of the muscle as you move. At both ends of the muscle belly, where it attaches to bone via tendons, lie more stretch receptors known as Golgi tendon organs (GTO). These limit excessive muscle contractions. As you start to stretch, a GTO sends a signal to the brain to resist the stretch and will prevent the muscle from overstretching or tearing.[5] This is why you should never force the body into a stretch; you are actually increasing the intensity of the system put in place to resist a stretch due to the contraction. Flowing yoga classes are perfectly designed to sneak past this system! To desensitize the protective stretch mechanisms, slowly work into each unpleasant pose with safe alignment and proper support from someone who knows how to prepare your body.

How Yoga Conquers Fear

One underlying limitation that often goes hand in hand with resistance during a stretch is the mental barrier we use to stop ourselves when we feel discomfort. Learning to identify the difference between mental and physical discomfort is one of the most unique gifts that stretching through yoga can offer. When I first started practicing yoga, I knew there were going to be limits. I had torn my hip labrum playing soccer in college and assumed that I'd have hip pain and poor motion in that joint forever. Before every class, I would tell the instructor, "This is my bad hip that doesn't bend well," so they wouldn't come over to push me into pigeon pose. Pigeon pose was the bane of my existence because I could feel discomfort in the exact area where I had had pain before the surgery. I convinced myself that because of the discomfort, it was a sign from my body that I was pushing too far and that I must be reinjuring the area. I avoided any deep hip poses that could pinch my hip capsule for about two years, and looking back now, I missed so much time for growth and progress. Once I received the correct physical treatment and found the emotional support needed to break that mental barrier, I was ready to face my fears and move past self-given limitations. You truly cannot progress in yoga or life if you avoid the uncomfortable positions—period.

In the presence of unstable or misaligned joints, the subconscious body will limit joint mobility. *Joint centration* is a term that describes the perfect position for a joint to be placed in so that the supporting muscles are evenly centered around the joint and can then fire together in unison. This safe contraction holds the articulating bone perfectly in place and makes it super stable.

When a bone is not sitting correctly in a joint socket, muscle imbalances are created, resulting in an altered range of motion. When trying to improve a joint's mobility, you cannot push it past a joint limitation if the body does not feel structurally supported. If the involved muscles are not firing properly and can't stabilize the joint correctly, they will never fully release to allow you to move in a direction that leads to injury. Once the mechanics supporting a joint are restored and properly stabilized, the flexibility of the surrounding muscles can be accessed then trained to become more flexible.

I find that many people come to yoga after an injury or while healing from a surgery. Learning yoga with the fear of injury or reinjury is a hard journey to tackle alone. If you remember from chapter 2, *psychosomatic pain* is a term used to describe how mental processes can result as a physical symptom even when a physical ailment or condition is not present. The limbic system in the brain remembers movements by closely intertwining the motor patterns together with the memory of how the movement feels emotionally. When emotional memories of previously painful movements are stirred and brought to the surface from the subconscious body, you will feel an old pain or unresolved injury.

I work with this type of patient in one-on-one private yoga sessions to have enough time to address the mental and physical limitations to movement, not something you'll collectively find in one doctor's visit. The biomechanical actions of our conscious brain can influence our unconscious reactions. Stretching elicits a release of neuroendocrine factors, such as endorphins, into the bloodstream. Endorphins go through the body to find receptors on the surfaces of cells within the central nervous system that will trigger relaxation and a good feeling, what yoga should feel like. To me, real yoga is going through the cycle of human emotions to reach the rewarding and satisfying sensation of progress, success, and self-control.

Honoring Your Current Limitations

Pain is inevitable; Suffering is optional.
— Buddhist proverb

When the body is pushed past a safe limit, injury ensues. After the onset of acute pain, the conscious mind is filled with immediate regret and creates memories of this new injury—how it began, the red flags leading up to the main event, and what turmoil it has caused following the injury. After a pain memory is filed, the brain has a fast pass to access the file if it feels you are recreating the same movement that led to the first encounter. When the body senses tissue damage and transmits pain signals to the cortex of the brain, the body experiences *nociception,* or pain signals.[7]

The structures surrounding a joint, such as capsular ligaments, intervertebral discs, or even blood vessels, have nerves that can experience and report nociception if irritated by extreme temperature, inflammation, or mechanical movement.[8] Receptors within the involved joints alert the alarm system within your brain, "She's going to try to bend again!" And if a threat to reinjury presents itself, the brain acts fast, locking down muscle units or joint range of motion to prevent excess movement. This self-defense routine is necessary to prevent injury but can exhaust the sympathetic nervous system (SNS) if constantly called to action (Review Chapter 3). Repetitive stressful triggers take away from the benefits of yoga, which aims to restore the parasympathetic nervous system and calm the mind-body connection.

So now what? You've gone too far and were hurt, making it time to seek the proper treatment that will expedite healing processes and minimize permanent damage. Once you're injured, try not to fall into the immediate downward spiral of devastation. It may not happen immediately, but you'll have to forgive yourself for the accident or disconnect of intuition. Having grace for your own mistakes is a vital component to moving forward and enables you to better receive the gift of healing hands. Find a provider who will intuitively guide you through the memory of an injury so that the mechanism will not produce a fear-avoidance pattern in future movement.

That mentality work is the key to a full recovery, but the physiological portion of healing cannot be ignored. Why? Because the ligaments that connect one bone to another bone at a joint unfortunately never fully restore their initial strength once they've been injured. The aftermath of healing creates scar tissue and disorganized collagen fibers, which alter the function of the ligamentous support system. Ligaments have a harder time bouncing back compared to the healing of muscles and tendons. Tendons connect one muscle to another bone, and after an injury, they heal slowly due to the progressive nature of their deterioration. A *tendinopathy* (the breakdown of collagen in a tendon) is usually the result of continuous forces that degenerate the tendon and its nutrient supply, as opposed to the harsh blow of a single incident.[7]

If muscle fibers are ruptured or torn in an explosive incident, the tissue elasticity in that local muscle belly may never return to normal. But with a muscle strain, the fibers can retract and return to their strong ability to contract while lengthening (what happens in the hamstrings as you bend forward). For yoga practitioners, muscle pulls may take a while to feel normal due to the nature of most poses. The asanas of yoga are a combination of concentric muscle contractions (muscles used to start the motion while shortening) and eccentric muscle contractions (muscles used to resist and stretch while lengthening). Yoga instructor Moises Aguilar puts it very simply, "Yoga is so freaking hard because you are using the same muscles to create a motion that you are also trying to stretch." The more aware you become during yoga practices, the more conscious control you will gain over this synchronized phenomenon. Then with proper soft tissue therapies and skeletal alignments, the body can withstand dynamic forces and offer the structural support needed to reaffirm mental healing.

Basic exercise physiology states that the body adapts to the demands placed on it. Just like building muscle tissue during strength training, small micro-tears of the muscle fibers are necessary to improve the flexibility of joint tissue and build bigger muscle cells. Basically, the active strain and healing process that we experience in a yoga class will slowly alter the tissue in our body to function throughout movement. Not in a few days' time of course, but over a long period of consistent and regimented practice. Annie O'Connor explains, "Increasing stress to scar tissue will ensure appropriate tensile stresses are applied to the joint for future resistance preparation."

The remodeling phase of healing can take from twenty-one days to over a year after an actual injury but understand that the soreness you feel after a yoga class is your body repairing the tissue from microtraumas you created from deep stretching.[7] This is why beginners should avoid buying that "ten days of unlimited yoga" plan. You will be sore, and at a certain point, continuously stretching the fibers that don't have time to heal in between classes can create weakness and vulnerability toward injury. Start at a slow and moderate frequency until you no longer experience heavy soreness from class. Then challenge yourself to more advanced poses or higher frequency of classes, building your stamina and yoga endurance.

Take a Breath

> Breathing attentively is yoga.
> Complete absorption in your work is yoga.
> Thinking about others instead
> of yourself is yoga.
> Anything which makes you
> forget your small self
> and become one with the infinite is yoga.
> — Karan Bajaj

One of the most powerful features of a properly moving spine is breathing restoration. Breathing is the key link to unlocking optimal neurology and is a large indicator of internal stress. Effortless breathing belongs to the unburdened and carefree human. By incorporating breath during movement reeducation, it serves as a control-alt-delete button to reset stress, tight muscles, and poor posture. The increase in neurological awareness that follows a spinal manipulation in chiropractic care allows the lungs and diaphragm to sync together. When restrictions between the spine and the ribs are released, the breathing apparatus can fully expand to provide your body with more fuel, which calms the primitive brain.

We tend to deplete our oxygen intake during times of tension, grief, or fear, which deprives the brain of a vital resource. Yoga offers each student an opportunity to witness the range between shallow, limited breathing and a fulfilling, free air exchange. The most efficient and powerful way to receive the benefits of yoga is to combine breathing with each movement. Most teachers offer breathing clues in a class, such as "Inhale, hold it at the top, and let it out." Each cue is meant to enhance the brain's connection with movement, stabilize certain joints, and ultimately, train the nervous system how to coordinate numerous systems at once.

There are many diseases and conditions that are understood to be influenced by breathing because the rhythmic core massage that breath produces can improve digestion and eliminate waste from the body. Accelerated by the nervous system's control of contracting and relaxing muscles, increased breathing encourages the heart to pump highly oxygenated blood throughout the body to stimulate cell metabolism. As the flow of one organ system improves from the influence of breath, other dependent organs come to life in response to new fuel, like the filtering system within the kidney, spleen, and liver.

Pranayama, the fourth limb of yoga philosophy, is the study of breath and its role as the bridge between the physical human and nonphysical experience. To the science community, the autonomic nervous system (ANS) controls what lies beneath our visible frame, home to the subconscious body. Pranayama's goal within yoga practices is to purify both the gross (visible) and subtle (invisible) systems of the body. The anatomical regions within the body that quickly demonstrate both our physical and emotional state are the diaphragms.

Ease the Pressure

A *functional diaphragm* is a term that I use to express a collection of muscles or flexible joints that are located within our cylindrical body in horizontal stacks. Each level of a functional diaphragm will act as a pump to inspire things like air or cerebral spinal fluid to move throughout the cavities of the body. When properly synchronized, the muscles of the diaphragms contract to stabilize joints and build compartments of pressurized, empty space between organs. When the skeletal system is aligned and properly moving, our amazing body knows how to use air cavities to support strong movement and sustain endurance postures.

The most popular diaphragm, commonly referred to in yoga classes but minimally understood, is the thoracic, or *respiratory diaphragm*. This muscle is called the diaphragm because it acts like a partition between cavities of the upper and lower torso. It lives inside the lower ribcage, just below the lungs, to aid in both expansion of breath and exhalation. When this primary breathing muscle is restricted or frozen due to injury, poor posture, or emotional stress, it is unable to function properly and we notice surface levels of breath limitation.[9] The challenge then, is identifying which trigger came first, the anxiety or the shallow breathing? Any inhibition in the thoracic diaphragm alerts the nervous system of a threat to successful breathing, which makes us feel unstable, anxious, and tired.[10]

While listening to years of vulnerable confessions on my table, it is hard to ignore the relationship between imbalanced or painful regions of the body and the emotional distress that the patient is experiencing. I would think, *of course they have a headache. All the pressure of life is weighing on their conscience without taking any steps toward action.* The helpless feeling of stagnation can be debilitating, and emotional pressure strains the body in the same way that physical pressure does; an aligned framework is essential for evenly distributing forces throughout the body. Any region that holds excessive weight without the support of surrounding aid is susceptible to fatigue and early degeneration.

My goal for discussing functional diaphragms is to highlight the necessity of a synchronized diaphragm system for both movement and general medicine. Author Bruno Bordoni said it best in his research on the body's continuity, "The diaphragm muscle should not be seen as a segment but as part of a body system." Within chiropractic care and yoga rehabilitation, I aim to restore the diaphragm groups of the musculoskeletal body, including the thoracic diaphragm, the perineum (pelvic floor), and the sphenobasilar joint (inside the skull). If pain resides in the hips for example, I analyze the health of all the levels of diaphragmatic movement to ease the load placed on the hips and the closest diaphragm (the perineum). By improving diaphragm continuity, we experience core involvement, spinal uprighting, and efficient muscle activation. This enables coordinated limb movement (safe aging) and athletic optimization (sustainable movement).[11]

Yogis claim that at least five of the anatomical diaphragms correlate with a subtle region of the energetic body (most lean toward seven). I witnessed this connection during a seminar where the chiropractor teaching had no intention of demonstrating anything beyond anatomic regions of the body that help support our core alignment. He shared an animated video of how diaphragms sync with our breath and the levels at which each lives along the spine. When the stacking diaphragms were individually highlighted along the axis of the body in the clip, my mouth fell open. The diaphragm levels, which are located near large collections of nerve bundles, were drawn exactly like the depiction of chakras (see image 9). I desperately scanned the room to see if anyone else was making the connection, until finally I locked eyes with a male student in the back row who was smiling from ear to ear—metaphorically speaking that is; his real ears were hidden beneath his dreadlocks. I thought, *Of course, the guy who never wears shoes knows about the chakras of yoga.* Despite our differences in appearance, our mission was the same. As the presenter moved on, we silently acknowledged that none of the respected doctors around us would look deep enough into their patients to accept that a relationship existed between the physical and subtle bodies. I knew that these diaphragms were portals to where true healing lies.

The Chakras of Yoga

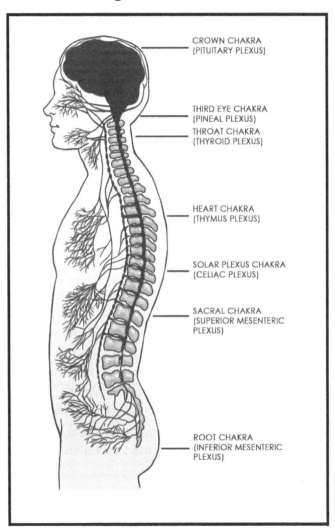

According to yogic philosophy, all humans have an energetic life force within them, known as prana. The current of prana is constantly flowing through minor spiraling channels of the body and then communicates through major meeting points, called chakras. This successful movement of this life force, like the meridians of Chinese Medicine, is a representation of our emotional state and subconscious health. A chakra is often depicted as a circulating wheel of petals aligned with the central axis of the body, representing the major seven powerhouses of energy (see image 9). Energy medicine teaches that the major seven chakras run along the spine starting at the base of the tailbone and numerically develop toward the apex of the skull, one through seven.

I honor the spiritual representations of chakras throughout many different philosophies, but my original interest in their existence revolved around their electric potential in our physical body. I think back to my cadaver days and how carefully we dissected layers of tissue around the spine. I don't remember stumbling upon glowing balls of tissue proving the existence of chakras, but we certainly weren't asked to look for those signs of intelligent life (long after someone's light has gone out). Separating nerves from the surrounding muscle or fatty tissue is incredibly difficult. My novice hands would never have been able to preserve the weblike structures of a nerve plexus where the main seven chakras have been described, but I could identify vital glands within the brain, neck, and abdomen. Anatomical charts accurately label important glands and nerve plexuses where yoga philosophy (that views the body as a vibrating, electrical, and deep-layered being) believes that each of the seven major centers lie within the body. The pituitary gland, the pineal gland, the thymus, and the adrenal glands are some of the contributors thought to correlate between both worlds of thought. Could the function of these glands and the nerves that regulate them be influenced by categories of emotions?

Reiki practitioners and the modern yoga community have developed a system of healing techniques that addresses each of the major chakra centers to align or restore their healing vibrations. Common emotions and themes have been categorized under the umbrella of each chakra that are thought to directly demonstrate the health of that energy center and its coordinating gland. For example, someone suffering from grief or abandonment may also have an imbalance in the heart chakra, leading to physical dysfunctions in the chest or thymus gland (chest pain, loss of appetite, weak posture, and decreased immune function).

The Ascension of Chakras

The healing practitioners who incorporate chakra balancing into their art believe that the chakras follow an upward journey toward evolution or enlightenment. Humans begin our electrical life complete with the necessary chakras, yet only through self-inquiry, life experience, and understanding can we gain access to their individual gifts. The gifts of neuroplasticity and self-awareness allow our species to develop past the unaware, dependent children who live to obtain primitive needs such as food, comfort, and familial relationships (themes of the first and second chakras). As we find safe avenues to develop past our primitive instincts, the base chakras progress alongside our emotional and spiritual development, which leads to free will (third chakra, solar), interpersonal relationships (fourth chakra, heart), creation of a personal identity (fifth chakra, throat), and ultimately a connection with the divine (seventh chakra, crown). Through the lenses of both a clinician and a healer, I'll introduce each of the major seven chakras, their affiliated themes of emotion, and how this ancillary outlook of the body can enhance your self-healing capabilities as you become a better version of yourself.

One (root chakra). The theme of the root chakra focuses on how medical intuitive Caroline Myss describes the needs of "one-self." These primitive needs satisfy the search of a low-functioning newborn and then stay with us throughout life. We will always thrive in a temperate climate that provides food in plenty, parental care and guidance, tribal acceptance, financial security, and physical safety. The root chakra communicates properly with other areas of the body when these foundational values are met. As adults, our willingness to provide ourselves with these needs will create a firm foundation in which we can fall back on or build from. Satisfying the necessities of the human experience paves the way for a fulfilled, nourished life, at any age. Someone who is struggling with these themes in life may experience tailbone pain, chronic low back pain, or pelvic floor disruptions. It is associated with the inferior mesenteric plexus and the glands of the reproductive system.

Two (sacral chakra). As a child ages, they start to develop a sense of self that is separate from their parents. Meaning, "Mom is there, yet I am here." "Mom can be distant from me and provide me with what I need." These interpersonal realities grow to match the challenges of each age group while refining external relationships, expressions of creative outlets, family dynamics, and the role you play in each of those settings. A properly nourished second chakra, situated in the center of the pelvis's sacral plexus, allows a person to seek family comforts like procreation and sharing physical aspects of life with other people. This perception of *one another* pushes us to gather the proper resources that will satisfy our human need to create something (like an actual human, a book baby, or a business, etc.) Those resources are almost always externally sourced, encouraging us to socially interact and utilize the complementary exchange of relationships. This creative center wants to express our togetherness while still depending on the personal values created during the root chakra stage of development. Challenges with the themes of the sacral plexus may manifest as a disruption in normal reproductive functioning, sacral or hip pain, or chronic urinary tract irritation. It is associated with the superior mesenteric plexus and the glands of the digestive system, such as the pancreas.

Three (solar plexus chakra). The third chakra surrounds the solar or celiac plexus and is an area that we metaphorically dedicate our sense of intuition and gut instinct to. Most of my patients call this region of the body their "core" and are aware that this needs to be a strong house that can support the rest of the body's activities. The same holds true for the energetic values of the chakra at this level; it resonates with the personality of someone who feels independent, brave, and trustworthy. The themes of a developing third chakra represent the blossoming of a teenager who, through trial and error, learns the values of discipline, risk management, and handling small crises. Like young adults, we build confidence based on the success of new projects, relationships, or accelerating accolades. Without identifying the outlets in life that have yet to solidify, the shaky foundation of the first two chakras will prevent someone from ascending past the values of the third chakra into higher forms of relationships and communication. It is never too late to lay down new values and attract a support system that complements this climb. Metaphysical pain that is associated with an imbalance in the solar plexus includes gastrointestinal disturbances, eating disorders, fluctuating weight, or adrenal fatigue.

Four (heart chakra). The connection between the lower and higher energy centers lands at the heart center, our fourth chakra. This area is associated with the cardiac plexus and the thymus gland. Of any region in the body, the heart has always been readily accepted as a sight of metaphorical pain. Art, music, and stories passed through generations always include someone who has "died of a broken heart" or "wears their heart on their sleeve." Why can we easily accept that our heart can be affected by stress or emotions but think the rest of the body is immune to the influence of similar triggers? The heart chakra and its affiliated physical attributes develop fully when a young adult begins to focus on the feelings of their inner world instead of the youthful distractions of the external world. While we demonstrate a love language at every age, the skills of the fourth chakra will mold into a permanent focal point for all the other talkative chakras to channel from. Yoga teaches that this region will not open without the healthy development of lower chakras, yet it may not have a way to communicate daily emotions without the aid of higher chakras. Suffering from an imbalanced fourth chakra can halt the communication and success of all the other regions, resulting in apathy, a rigid mid spine, and shortness of breath. Living in alignment with your true purpose allows this area to flourish. Like I shared earlier in this section, someone suffering from heart wrenching emotions can experience physical dysfunctions in the chest or thymus gland which has an important role in immunity.

Five (throat chakra). The fifth chakra emanates from the region of the thyroid gland, which is situated just north of the vocal cords. Pivotal functions such as hormone regulation, sound production, digestion, and respiration take place at this level of our human form, which correlates with the importance of the throat chakra. In yoga philosophy, this energetic center is the representation of an adult's maturation of will. The symbolism of a healthy, flexible neck portrays someone who respects their power of choice. Affirming our truths with a *yes* or *no* will leave an imprint on the physical body that influences those we encounter. Someone who struggles with clear communication, self-expression, or identities may also experience physical disruptions in the throat, thyroid, neck, or mouth. As a chiropractor, I frequently combine adjustments to the cervical spine (neck) with audible affirmations to demonstrate the influence that loving words have over pain near this region. With the input from balanced lower chakras, the fifth chakra is an amazing outlet to express gratitude through dialogue, singing, or chanting.

Six (third eye chakra). The third eye is a symbol that is presented in many Eastern cultures as an intuitive region of the mind's eye where humans can access gifts or heightened senses. Medically, the location of the third eye has been pinned to the pineal gland within the brain, which is notorious for its mysterious functions. We do not fully understand this gland but know that it plays a role in hormone production, light interpretation (melatonin regulation), and can influence the functions of the entire body in response to increasing light or decreasing light. Our mood, cravings, and fatigue levels are all monitored by this brain center which is why headaches, light sensitivity, and insomnia may all be related to an imbalanced sixth chakra. Developing an awareness of this region helps the conscious adult perceive experiences and opportunities in a different "light." What once was the focus of a narrow-minded teen is now the observation of a broad-spectrum adult who takes others' points of view into consideration while developing their own values. The conscious individual who openly recruits this chakra can seek truths that are detached from social or cultural norms. Most yoga teachers speak to this area of the body when inviting the class to use their *drishti,* or concentrated gaze. An accepting adult uses the gifts of this intentional gaze to witness more than their own routines or challenges.

Seven (crown chakra). The seventh of the major chakras is drawn at the apex of the central nervous system. Despite the name of the crown (which most relate to the crown of the skull), this energy center is dedicated to the functions of the pituitary gland within the brain. This crowning gland orchestrates most of the hormone production throughout the rest of the body and beautifully represents the need for connection in our life. As an aging adult gracefully reviews their role on earth, they often come to terms with a higher power and divine plan. This energy center demonstrates the final ascension we make toward unity with the unknown and fulfills the absence of meaning or purpose that earthly possessions could not satisfy. Chronic imbalances in the pituitary gland affect the entire body and, through the eyes of an energy healer, can manifest in neurological disorders. They believe the crown of the body is the main site of electric conduction. Someone who struggles to access the crown chakra may feel isolated, lost, and fearful each day. By deeply connecting with the physical sensations of movement, breathing, and pain relief, I help each patient restore their faith in the human experience. Once they leave my care, I hope they feel ready to look for spiritual or emotional guidance. The practices within yoga that best develop and utilize this chakra are the many forms of meditation or prayer.

Interpreting Chakra Involvement during Medical Care

One of the most valuable gifts I received from working with patients in America's Bible Belt was to witness the power of belief. I never expected to find such a culturally and spiritually diverse population flow through my office in Tulsa, Oklahoma, but I soon realized that no matter how much science or medical referrals I offered certain patients, they still chalked their recovery up to faith and their relationship with a higher power. As an observant witness who struggled with healing the faithful, I have seen patients with pain disappear immediately and joint function restore completely without any of my intervention. Can I blame the remission on subconscious truths or external sources of spiritual aid? We will never know for sure, but one thing is undeniably sure: never underestimate the power that someone places on their beliefs.

With chakras specifically, many of my patients believe that their physical symptoms are information sent from the conversing chakras deep within their subtle body. As an intuitive healer, I will support their beliefs to the fullest if they improve and are not avoiding any medically necessary interventions. As a manual therapist, I try to keep the themes of the chakras in the back of my mind as I develop a relationship with each patient. Someone who is not responding from manual care but expresses the pain of their divorce in every visit may not be someone who I can truthfully help at a structural level until the contents of their emotional heart have been resolved. Referrals and "prescriptions" for mindful activities may be the best thing I can offer someone during the healing process. Inspired by the themes of the chakras, I've listed simple questions below that a provider can use to spark self-inquiry and healing realizations while treating. It is amazing how differently we each respond to those questions, and some of the answers have revealed medical information that the patient may not have ever disclosed otherwise, giving new life to the existing care plan.

1. During the time that this pain started, was there a big change happening in your life?

2. What do you do to nurture yourself?

3. What part of your body do you trust the most?

4. What leads most of your decision-making—your brain, heart, or gut?

5. Who can you ask for help from without any guilt or filtering?

6. How long do you foresee this injury lasting?

7. What do you think your body (mental, emotional, physical) is telling you that it needs?

The Healing Hands of Yoga

A common supplement to popular yoga classes that has not yet been discussed is the benefits of a *mudra*. A mudra is a collective of positions that accompany meditative postures or the asanas (poses) of yoga. Take a moment to look up some examples. Easily recognized in classic models of Christian saints, Hindu gods, and Buddhist figurines, the gestures of the healing hands, when aligned with the intention to manifest a specific benefit, offer the practitioner a super charge. The hands have always been an outward representation of our inner desires and dialogue.

Modern yoga philosophy teaches a variety of mudras that can be added to a pose, igniting specific intentions, such as obtaining knowledge or expressing gratitude. Defined by the shape of the hands or a symbol that the paired fingers create, the hands are thought to activate chakra centers and cultivate energy (which is also the aim of qigong in Chinese medicine). Through the eyes of my acupuncture training, I see a correlation between the stimulation points of a mudra and the meridian lines of the hand. Touching the acupuncture points with a focus on healing that organ will realign certain elements of the body, such as metabolism (fire), filtration (water), breath (air), and fertility (earth). Chiropractic philosophy has always demonstrated the healing power that hands have when in the right position, so implementing mudras into my yoga practice was a welcome addition.

To bring the benefit of mudras to my patients in the office, I recommend keeping it simple. Look for opportunities to bring awareness to the patient's hands while working on distant regions of the body. For instance, while working on knee pain, are the patient's hands clenched into fists? Maybe recommend that they touch the hurt region with you as you assess what needs to be done. Or, while a patient lies on their back, instead of letting the nervous system maintain a defensive posture, ask the patient to uncross their arms and intentionally place the palms in a position that will make them comfortable. I offer placing one hand on the heart and one hand on the solar plexus if the patient displays a need to reconnect with their body. For some, open palms facing the ceiling or sky help place the subconscious mind in a position that can better receive healing or nourishment.

The influence of yoga will reach every cell in your body's chemistry. The masters who dedicated their life to advancing the practices of yoga made sure to include every aspect of the mind, body, and spirit in their teachings to offer something complete to students. Beyond strength, flexibility, and focus, there are ascending themes of a yoga class to accelerate or heighten the experience. We discussed the foundations of breath and its ability to synchronize the entire physical body. Chapter 5 also introduced the benefits of vibrations and how sounds throughout a yoga class can stimulate both the physical structure and its energetic components. For all that yoga has to offer—movements, breathing, inquiry, energy, mudras—there are no set rules, only suggestions and practiced templates that others have found beneficial along their journey upward.

Yoga Review Questions

1. What is a physical limitation you believe to be true about your body?

   a. (e.g., I can't run because I have arthritis in my knees.)

2. What is an emotional limitation you believe to be true within your body?

   a. (e.g., I can't socialize because I have depression.)

3. What is a mental limitation you have in your mind about your body's capabilities?

   a. (e.g., I am going to end up with dementia like my mother did.)

4. What outlet of movement do you use to prove those limitations aren't permanent or true?

5. Have you tried yoga before? If so, was it the correct environment for you and your goals?

6. Build the perfect studio or yoga practice for your needs:

   a. studio: (proximity/size/decorations/price)
   b. community: (population most likely to attend)
   c. style: (techniques taught/philosophy vs. exercise based)
   d. interactions: (intimate and hands-on vs. offers space and isn't pushy)
   e. offerings: (private sessions/workshops/group study, etc.)

7. Identify your biggest limitations to creating a regular yoga practice.

    a. (Finances, time, support, conflicting ideologies, injury, etc.)

8. What will keep you compliant with yoga?

Like ripples on the water,
every gift returns to the giver.
What we affirm in others,
we actually affirm in ourselves.
— Deepak Chopra

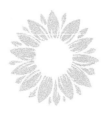

CHAPTER 7

Intention and Mental Dialogue

Healing Insight—The Mentality of I Am Affirmations

I was fortunate enough to grow up in a family that lived by the phrase "What you tell your brain, your brain tells your body." It took me many years to discover and study the science behind this advice, but I was happy to learn from a young age that attitudes of thought directly affect your body and its performance. Thanks to the alternative nature of my clinical experience, I have zero doubt about the power your mind has over health and why affirmations play such a large role in that transformation. An *affirmation* is most often witnessed in the form of an oath or a law, but on a personal level, it is an audible belief that expels your mental attitude, "I am healing" or "I am accepted." The conviction associated with an affirmation helps to relay truth, honesty, and loyalty to whomever hears it. The "mantras" are repetitive affirmations that many healers use in yoga classes and therapy sessions to seal the progress made during a self-inquiry practice.

This self-promise calls forward the attention of Carl Jung's *total psyche* (a combination of both the ego and the unconscious self) to agree on a quality you hold within. The declaration of "I am ..." is a brave and fear-conquering statement that speaks that attribute into existence. The intention that resonates behind an affirmation is as powerful as its level of truth. All truth is spoken from a place in the body that feels safe, knows love, and hopes to spread it. This emotional vibration resonates through words, emitting a high vibrational frequency into the world to accelerate the positive reaction. Like a radio frequency, we are each an antenna that sends out sound to match what we long to create. "Something" receives the transmission and responds, which is a phenomenon called manifestation. Without truth in the statement, the effect is weaker. Saying, "I am rich," does not magically create wealth, especially if you are focusing on a lacking sense of finances and do not believe the statement is true. Knowing your worth from a state of deep truth will attract more wealth into your life but doubt and concerns of materialism often cloud the truth of statements in this category.

Affirmations are the initial stamping of an acknowledgment on our souls that we will then wear as we walk through life, emanating a positive influence over everything we interact with. In my personal and professional practice, I like to break down the pieces of an affirmation statement and why as human beings we hold the significance of our identity to the highest standards.

"I"

A child begins to recognize themselves as a "self" by the age of two, no longer combined with the existence of the mother. Then begins the process of developing how they think about themselves from the perspective of a second person, which we will spend a lifetime developing. The complex, overlapping roles of self-concept and our place in society will continue to unfold in time, but that initial epiphany of *I* never leaves. We place so much importance on the influence of *I*, often confusing the difference between *I* and our name. On the surface, *I* represents your titles, documented name, and what values those represent to the world.

As a dramatic example, in the famous play *The Crucible,* John Proctor battles with his conscience when he is persuaded into a false confession that will commit many innocent people to their death, saving himself as a result. He goes along with the confession to witchcraft until he must sign his name and decides against living with the guilt of his signature's repercussion. He cries, "Because it is my name! Because I cannot have another in my life! ... How may I live without my name? I have given you my soul; leave me my name!" Overlooking his obsession to maintain a good reputation, we can all relate to his battle of questioning what his name stands for and what about his identity is important. In my treating sessions, I'll describe the *I* in an affirmation as the unshakable, authentic, nontitle, and nonidentity part of you. While I am a daughter, a doctor, and a woman, when speaking in terms of an affirmation, the *I* goes beyond those roles.

Rebecca Campbell, author of *Rise Sister Rise,* calls this authentic portion of self "the part of you that is timeless and knows exactly what lights it up. The part of you that is waiting for you to remember, to discover, to unlock, and set it free." Developing the depths of *I* will be a continuous journey of solidifying what you learn about your beliefs. As soon as that picture forms, we are asked to conquer the fear of letting that I change. As soon as we identify with a label, we are limited to societal and personal definitions of that title, which comes with how we should act or interact. Developing your I should set you free, not switch you into a new realm of captivity. Utilizing what gifts you possess, work to build a flowing form of *I* that is beyond titles and external experiences.

"I Am"

The second portion of the affirmation equation is the ownership of the I—understanding what *I* is and allowing it to sink into your full being. *I am* should be understood by its values, not by its semantics in the English language, because we are one of the few languages that uses the adjective to identify ourselves instead of identifying a current state of our existence. In Spanish, for example, *I am* can be a possessive phrase used to describe how a noun or abstract noun can belong to a person or be felt by a person; I have hunger or I am in possession of hunger, "Tengo hambre." In Spanish, stating, "I am hunger," as an English-speaking person does, "Estoy hambre," states a drastic state of near starvation. The unique adjective in the English language states, "I am hungry," as if we are identified by the feeling or sensation. This identity with our emotions or experiences, when applied to greater adjectives, denotes a permanence and attachment to things that dictate our future perception, such as "I am diabetic" or "I am depressed." We have the option to choose "I have diabetes" or "I am currently suffering with depression" but tend to skip the hassle and affirm those identities into our being by stating *I am* ....

The *am* of an affirmation is about ownership and aligning with the state of authentic offerings that were acknowledged by the *I,* so use its power for positive and healthy language only. We proudly and unconditionally take ownership for things our values or morals dictate as worthy. If your timeless sense of *I* feels beautiful, then by stating, "I am beautiful," you are owning that truth and believing that you can emanate that feeling for every living thing to see. With this deep understanding of an affirmation, it should not matter what comes after *I am* because you truly know what the first two words represent. We all need reminders in times of doubt, which is why the third word helps direct the affirmation toward manifestation.

For example, the powerful statement of "I am free" creates amazing physical results in pain relief and emotional clarity. When my patients mentally create an ideal environment for freedom, voice their need for it, and believe that it can be obtained, I watch how this declaration of emotional, physical, and spiritual independence washes over them. Freedom is so much more than the conflict between captivity or liberation. As Viktor Frankl discovered in *Man's Search for Meaning,* freedom is a choice, a permission to move, as well as the strength to forgive someone who hurt you. Freedom is a chance to rewrite, rewire, and realign with your authentic perception of a healthy life. So much meaning can pack into three vibrational words. Those vibrations will shake off false beliefs before transmuting into healing waves of life source.

Throughout this chapter, I will explain how the mental perception of our bodies and the subconscious dialogue we unknowingly participate in are influenced by factors that lie deep in the brain. Academics and clinicians accept the power of the subconscious mind now more than ever, recognizing how the intelligent brain not only interprets but then enhances sensory data to match our personal values. This process of imaginative reasoning often creates an artificial transmission of filtered information to our conscious mind. By understanding the motivation for detrimental perceptions, you can reverse the effects and find the appropriate healing affirmation.

Connecting with Affirmations

My favorite affirmation is an all-encompassing prayer to acknowledge my singular existence in a void of eternity. By recognizing that everything is everything, nowhere is somewhere, and that we are all in the same boat, I have used this affirmation time and time again to bring my chaotic soul back to earth.

"I am everyone, I am everything, I am everywhere."

"I Am Everyone"

> Dedicating our lives to serving the world
> connects us to one another and reminds us to
> focus on something bigger than ourselves.
> — Lisa Rankin, *The Fear Cure*

I am is an energetic frequency that aligns the cellular levels of both physical and electrical processes in your body. This powerfully transformative vibration wakes up the signaling system in your physical body to alter or mend itself to match the image and state of mind that you are claiming. When you affirm, "I am calm," your brain has stored expectations of the definition of that word and stored memories of the reaction to the word; it knows how you feel when you are calm. Immediate hormones and neurotransmitters are released to send signals to your body to once again find that response and restore the desired sensation of calm to your senses. With that instant transfer of chemicals in mind, it should be no surprise that we can feel physical discomfort in the presence of someone sharing their challenges with us. Our brain can relate to most crises that other humans experience, and if not, it uses our senses to analyze the physical signs of the person we're communicating with to try to understand what it would feel like.

Say, "I am everyone," with the awareness of how many people you have longed to help or share feelings with in such a short life. I have met multiple heart-stopping and soul-touching humans who mirrored myself in many ways. I loved the parts of them that represented the best of me and learned to embody the strengths of those role models that I knew I didn't currently possess. I still hear the worries and struggles of countless people each day and can find myself in each of their stories, in each of their separate and seemingly distant lives. To comfort the people in my healing hands, I aim to reassure them that every other mother, daughter, son, and father has dealt with similar tribulations. I do not have to pretend that we have strength in numbers. I witness it every day. Such a simple statement can exclude every barrier of segregation—*I am everyone.*

"I Am Everywhere"

> Fleuris là où tu es plantée.
> Bloom where you are planted.
> — French saying

Before I was fully matured or conscious enough to speak with strangers, I kept to myself in social settings, which reinforced my growing fears that I was isolated and alone. It was not until I relocated across the country at twenty-three that I felt what true loneliness was. Hours from my family and friends, I studied alone, dropped my head in between classes, and ran by myself for nearly an entire year. This was around the time I suffered a severe soccer injury and would turn to yoga's medicine. Luckily, graduate programs have a way of bringing people together. I slowly created a circle of beautiful friends within my class that made my school experience joyful. Their support reinforced the understanding that moving forward, in the real working world, I'd have to grow into a socialite if I wanted to excel professionally.

After a year of practicing yoga at home, I got a job cleaning the bathrooms of a local power yoga studio. Each morning at five am, I mopped, brushed toilets, disinfected mats, and polished floors so I could afford to take classes before school started. At each yoga class that I attended, I challenged myself to start a conversation with at least two strangers at the studio. Yoga became the beautiful ice breaker that allowed me to develop a welcoming personality while meeting healthy, like-minded people. Not every interaction was ideal, but that exercise gifted me with rare opportunities to find myself or the culture that I missed within the lives of strangers. A simple greeting or compliment can unlock the door to a conversation that reveals similarities or insane coincidences. The warmth I felt from a shared experience could carry me for hours as if I was with my family and friends back east.

That healing energy occupied my mind through the words "*I am* everywhere." I am everywhere, in the sense that through shared activities, culture, and passions, we can be connected to our family from any point on the globe (or beyond). By celebrating the growth of those you care about, it is like you are experiencing their growth as well. Connect with others to spread the ripple and reach with impact in directions you would never reach by yourself. Your message and influence left on the lives of those you interact with will have an exponential effect on each soul they share that imprint with, and so on. *I am everywhere.*

"I Am Everything"

> There are a hundred thousand species of love,
> separately invented, each more
> ingenious than the last,
> and every one of them keeps making things.
> — Richard Powers, *The Overstory*

Say, "I am everything," as we acknowledge the depth of our unknown connection to living things that our bodies are influenced by on an energetic level. In the monotony of our daily routines, we walk past seemingly inanimate objects, unaware of the also aging plants or tiny animals around us. We share spaces with the living things to provide an inhabitable environment, equally giving and taking. When the balance tips, vulnerable lives cannot thrive.

All living cells vibrate to an unknown pacemaker and creator. All life ages better with the aid of high-vibrational nutrition, a safe location, and a communal network of support. No role is more important than another in an ecosystem, yet while looking at life through the microscope of your own needs, it's easy to forget that the planet does not revolve around "me." Many of my patients have shared that getting out in nature helps them to find a healthier order of priorities. Walk into the woods or stand next to an ocean; allow these awe-inspiring scenes to place your role on the planet into perspective, lessening the ego's frantic chatter. *I am everything* reminds us that there is nothing isolating about life on earth beyond our own mental barriers.

I Am Poem

Selfish soul work must be done
while learning to be everyone.
Seeing the likeness of yourself in
others delivers everyone.
Shared experiences open the mirror of
familiarity with everyone.

Losing yourself is vital to finding everywhere.
Loving another on the opposite side
of the world fuels everywhere.
Access to immediate, online
influence spreads everywhere.

Being moved by the timelessness of
an ancient tree is everything.
Exploring the chemistry between man
and sea tastes like everything.
Remembering our evolution with
creatures protects everything.

Developing What Is True

> Life experiences mirror our beliefs.
> — Louise Hay, *You Can Heal Your Life*

While defining affirmations, I mentioned that they have the greatest influence when you believe in the truth of the statement. So, what develops our truths? And is that a fluid concept? The perception we hold of the world and our role in it has an extraordinarily strong influence on our individual reality. *Reality*, meaning our outlook on existence, is built by the accumulation of our values and experiences that define our truths. It would be a rarity to find two people with an almost identical set of foundational values and supplementary experiences. Blended with the power of interpretation, the senses in our body create a personal reality, one that doctors, or healers try to quickly understand each time they interact with you.

Our perception is like a set of emotional lenses that we hold in our back pocket, ready to switch out with other pairs when we choose to. Leonard Mlodinow, a theoretical physicist, describes in his book about the mind's control of behaviors how "we accept visions concocted in the mind without question, not realizing they are a personal interpretation." Our view on life dictates what we focus on during each day, so we look for reinforcing sensory information to prove our story matches what's coming in.[1] For example, when you wake up in a bad mood and decide the rest of the day will likely follow suit, what happens? You can go through the rest of the day looking for other negative experiences to prove your mental story. It's possible though to observe that you are wearing clouded lenses, switch them out, and then begin to perceive the experiences of your day in a more positive light.

The Reticular Activating System

The connection between the information we receive from the body and where it lands in the brain has a lot to do with the reticular activating system (RAS). This group of nerves lives in the brain stem and serves as a security guard for messages sent from regions of the body as they travel toward higher brain centers. I was encouraged to remember this neuroanatomy in hopes that it would add scientific supplementation to my theories of why humans choose to perceive the world in a way that sustains painful or limiting physical abilities. I knew that the RAS acts like a filter to block unnecessary sensory information to the brain so that more important (or currently interesting) stimuli gets through. It seemed like a logical explanation for how the body could train itself to seek out reinforcing stimuli to support a current reality. I found myself passing on relevant information about the RAS during heart-to-hearts with patients that I'd heard from some other "very respected" references (self-help books, podcasts, inspirational speakers). "It's the part of the brain that looks for synchronicities such as repetitive numbers or a new word that you just learned."

If I was going to truly implement the concept that the RAS is responsible for increased recognition patterns and creating filters of perception, then I had to do my own review of research. I needed to better understand the physiology before comfortably using it in my work. After weeding out numerous articles about synchronicities and the law of attraction (all things I love to personally practice but cannot medically endorse), I found information on how the reticular activating system determines where our messages and resulting attention will be directed.

The RAS is named the ascending arousal system due to the direction of stimuli that alter and arouse the central nervous system. Among other sensory regulators, the RAS is constantly scanning incoming information, looking for first-class customers to expedite toward the brain, such as information from the eyes and pivotal organ systems. The brain is constantly bombarded with information in our surroundings and can't handle responding to them all simultaneously. To prioritize the information, the RAS helps you tune out daily noise that seems unthreatening or irrelevant to you. *Sensory gating* describes the filtering input and output that takes place at this region of the brain stem. It is the filtering process that intercepts ascending information and determines how important the message will be.[2]

The sensory gating mechanism aims to save space by not allowing conflicting messages to land in the brain before we've had time to process and respond appropriately on the surface. Have you ever zoned out on a loud bus while reading a book, only to snap out of it the moment someone calls you by name? Thank the RAS for working full-time underneath your awareness so you didn't miss your stop. The gating mechanism, like all systems in the body, can be upregulated or downregulated amid chemical or physical imbalances to search for homeostasis.

PTSD Protection

Although I can't claim that we have a conscious influence on what key words or emotions will influence the gating mechanism, some research has targeted specific populations of patients with a faulty RAS that could shed light on the theory. In the brain of someone with post-traumatic stress disorder (PTSD), the gating mechanism has been found to be upregulated, causing exaggerated and hyperreactive responses to sensory stimuli. This causes trouble sleeping, anxious preparation for perceived threats, and exposure to illogical triggers of the fight-or-flight system of nerves.[3]

I worked with Sharon as a virtual client during the pandemic. Sharon was seeking help from numerous providers when another chiropractor referred her to me. Among other physical imbalances, she was suffering from anxiety, insomnia, and other signs of PTSD. I knew she was divorced and currently sharing custody of her child who had special needs. With the added stress of quarantine, Sharon was drowning. After some guided movement and yogic breath training, we discussed how emotional pain was wreaking havoc inside her mind's body.

She had made a huge breakthrough recently by telling her previous husband that she needed more help with childcare. The father agreed and brought their daughter to his new home, where he lived with a new girlfriend and child. Sharon unfortunately found no relief in her daily routine or physical distress after making this healthy decision. She was now experiencing what I call a "no hangover." She said no, identifying her healthy boundaries, but was now feeling the hangover of guilt and shame afterward.

Each day, she admitted to looking for something about her behavior to blame, reaching back into her childhood for reasons to reinforce her perception of being *broken*. Through guided meditation, we brought Sharon through the visual of her daughter's upcoming birthday party, which would depict an event where the new members of her daughter's growing family would have to coexist, and each bring a gift to the party. By identifying the personal and intangible gifts that each person would present to her daughter, Sharon found a sense of relief. Realizing that loving support can come from sources outside herself, she was able to unload the burden of self-guilt she was holding from not raising her daughter alone.

As homework and self-study, we closed our session with the recommendation of researching the reticular activating system. I want all my patients and clients to believe that they are healing themselves, and with access to more understanding, we can accelerate that process. I briefly described the RAS to her and explained why I thought it relevant to her behavior of constantly seeking signs of "brokenness" in her life. She took to it immediately and smiled at the idea that a physiological program in her body, like all other healthy humans, was facilitating her negative perception. This inclusion gave her a sense of calm as she said, "Oh good. I'm not crazy." I encouraged her to use neurological mechanisms to empower her ability to choose healthier responses to stimuli and, by doing so, retrain her brain to allow positive messages through the gate alongside life-sustaining, primitive threats. Leave a kind, calm adult at the gate instead of entrusting a defensive and easily injured child to dictate our emotional behaviors.

Mirror Neurons

> Matter is a Mirror.
> — Don Miguel Ruiz, *The Four Agreements*

It is difficult not to revert to the fundamental behaviors we learned as children. Those memories were chiseled into the original blank slate of development and have since been layered over with Wite-out and updated by adult notes. Most of the original files were developed by *mirror neurons*. During scans of the brain, this class of neurons shows the same activity while the subject performs an action as it does when they observe another person performing the action.[4] Mirror neurons are considered imitation neurons that play a large role in young development.

Any parent can attest to witnessing the effects of mirror neurons and the amazement of watching a child mimic their gestures or actions such as eating. The same visuomotor neurons follow us through life and develop into an active member of our movement perceptions, our imitation of others body language. It is currently accepted that the term "intention understanding" describes how we process information when witnessing the action of another individual.[5] We initially see the action of another while simultaneously attempting to comprehend why or for what the movement is intended. The reticular activating system of ascending arousal is very involved in the process of intention understanding and more intimately tied with the perception of movement than previously thought.[2] It is essential in formulating our sensations associated with movement and can be evoked without ever completing the motion.

I would love to see more tailored research done on this area in regard to healing caused by mental imagery in hope that the results would shed light on our ability to absorb the pain of another. Within existing research, I did find that many studies argue that the mirror neuron system is involved in experiencing both emotions and empathy. Subjects who are self-reported as empathic proved to have stronger activations both in the mirror system for hand actions and the mirror system for emotions.[5] Similar results have been obtained for subjects who feel pain during the observation of a painful situation, mostly when the other person involved was a loved one. Taken together, these experiments suggest that feeling emotions is due to the activation of circuits that correspond with emotional responses. In short, cells in the brain appear to fire in similar patterns as the nervous system that they're watching.

I worked with a muscle testing doctor in 2018 while learning to comprehend energy medicine. He was a retired chiropractor but felt more like a therapist to me. I sought his care to stay in touch with reality as the magic on my table tried to drown my mind in a sea of questions. His work highlighted the filing system of our brain and the skewed stories we work to affirm in ourselves. One of our discussions landed on an early memory of mine in which I was reprimanded as a child for social awkwardness by my teacher. I was punished in school for being disruptive or asking questions outside of the material being covered that day. I thought my awareness of things unseen proved I was destined to be different from my peers or colleagues. He calmly responded to my story, "that's not an example of you having early signs of special gifts."

"Your earthly gift, the reason you are changing hidden things in your patients, is your gift of observation."

Limitations to Behavioral Change

> Every decision you make creates a ripple in
> the interconnected sea that joins all life;
> there is nothing too big or too small,
> every conscious act counts.
> — Rebecca Campbell, *Rise Sister Rise*

While living in an overlapping world between treating patients and evaluating my own life stories, I have witnessed how fear stems from the thought of making a wrong decision that will permanently influence a projected future path. That path, it seems, will let down an invisible sense of future potential. We can all feel the pull of something luring just out of reach, encouraging us to make calculated decisions toward progress. The anxiety and flighty behaviors of patients who find their way into my office are minimized by using a few simple organizational methods. I'm not a therapist, so I always encourage patients to continue seeking treatment outside the office, but on my table, we conquer fear using affirmations, the model of behavioral changes, and mindful movement to develop an awareness of the body's reaction to life's decisions.

Lay the Foundation for Fear

I frequently hear an expression that I learned in chiropractic school run through my head while treating patients, "You can't shoot a cannon off a canoe." In relation to the body, we use this to explain the importance of a strong core before exerting intense movements with the ankles or shoulders. I use the phrase for life experiences as well, especially when the conversation revolves around the crippling fear of making changes. You cannot ignite a big change in life from an unstable surface. Change—the cannonball—won't go far, and the boat of life will capsize if you're not careful. In the midst of transition or chaos, I remind patients to pull all their focus and worry back to what they can feel in the present, which is perfectly demonstrated by movement such as running or yoga. Once focused on the now and not dreading the future, they are able to put maximized efforts into building a firm foundation in at least one pillar of life.

This rock will be a home base for evolution if you are questioning your marriage, job, income, and health-care routine all at once. It is overwhelming to think of finding a way to change all aspects of life simultaneously, so find your rock and gently expand when things feel more stable. A rock can be a reliable person (or dog), comforting place, or soothing activity—one consistent piece of life that will travel with you throughout any season of change.

In my biggest transition of life, the first thing I had to create was a solid rock or home to call my own. This physical location would be a "launching pad for something great," according to my lovely Realtor. I worked hard and patiently waited until the universe helped me purchase my first home. Within my new healing space, I was comfortable enough to then grieve the loss of a relationship while having my daily chiropractic work to occupy my hands. This stage of beautiful growth ignited self-love and the chance to meet the right person for my future life. With the pillars of love and shelter in place, I could then answer the call to writing this guide, which would require most of the willpower that I had been offering daily to patients. I would never have taken the leap toward leaving such a good job without the growing phase of the first three steps. Although this process took just over one year, I constantly think back and congratulate my past self for being diligent and committing to the unknown. Maybe our future selves are to blame for the gut instinct we hear talking to us in the now? If so, thank you, solar plexus chakra, for keeping in touch with all versions of myself.

Fear, Meet Wonder

Amber Rae, author and motivational speaker, categorizes the two conversations inside our heads as "wonder and worry." Her definition of worry explains how doubt, fear, and belittling self-talk occur in the mind when addressing a potential change. The voice of the logical mind forces the body to make sensible decisions for a danger-free life. Decisions are limited by worry and reinforced by the only thing we can trust is certain, a previously lived experience. Based on prior experiences, deeply ingrained cycles of fear live in the brain to offer proof of what mistakes or discouraging decisions have created in the past. The brain remembers the uncomfortable sensation and pulls those chemical reactions to the surface as we flirt with wonder in the present time.

Wonder is the opposite dialogue, the soul voice of internal conversations that are not always logical. Wonder is the voice in the back of your head that refuses to be stifled—the visionary time spent creating hypothetical fantasies that question the limits of our greatest potential. With the right intention and manifestation, wonder can overpower worry and make room for growth. I believe that both worry and wonder are time dependent, so I encourage each patient to assign a timeline to their current stressors to identify when things started and how much longer they anticipate the strain to linger.

Timelines for Freedom

Big-picture thinkers can get overwhelmed by planning too far in advance. The gift of heightened awareness can also be a curse if someone projects their energetic effort outward in too many directions. In the midst of chaos, stay present and reel your energy in so it can nourish the body's immediate requests. Then with a completely focused mind, choose the next step of a healing journey. Life has a way of changing long-term plans in the blink of an eye, so create a flexible mindset to ensure that planning and preparation can adapt along the way. For the big-picture thinkers, I challenge you to draw a timeline for each of the issues you are dealing with. Be honest; place things on a scale between temporary and seemingly permanent. Ask yourself, "Will I truly be affected by this discomfort forever, or is this pressure going to alleviate soon?" This scale will allow you to prioritize where to place healing efforts. I suggest tackling the most temporary concerns first then, watch the momentum build. By creating a realistic timeline for change or struggle, you will break the cycle of dread that works to convince you that the current issue will perpetuate forever.

To the patients who are losing hope, I share the words of medical doctor and author Lisa Rankin, "As it turns out, the difference between optimists and pessimists lies in how permanent, pervasive, and personal they perceive good and bad events to be." She means that optimistic personalities are not naive in thinking that bad things can't happen; they believe that when things inevitably go wrong, it's just a small speed bump along the road toward growth. Pessimistic personalities witness the speed bump as yet another horrible life event that perpetuates a learned pattern of discouragement; the speed bumps reinforce their defeated outlook on life.

Most of the worry that we anticipate is mentally generated. The nervous brain places protective traps throughout the body and anxiously waits to receive sensations that prove our fear-driven theories. In the office, my role beyond pain relief is to help others understand their perception of what the future will bring or what the past "did" to their body. This liberation allows all attention to be placed on present successes. When they look to me for answers to their healing questions, I often tell them, "Let the present sensations be the response you are looking for." If pain can be altered by affirmations, positive imagery, or guided meditation, the priority issue cannot be dissected by medicine or structural intervention. The true language of the body is best felt during focused movement while the mind chooses to interact with a present stimulus. This is why yoga and meditation are such beautiful mediums for holistic healing; providers don't administer them to you. They invite you to fully participate throughout the therapies so that in time you are ready to take the climb yourself.

Brittany's Climb

I had the honor of meeting a young woman who was severely injured in a rock-climbing fall. Within the first year of opening its doors, her injury was the most severe accident that the local rock-climbing gym had seen. As a result, she became quite a legend within the member community. After free-falling from fifty-five feet, Brittany suffered a severely fractured ankle, numerous broken ribs, and a shattered vertebrae in her low back. While recovering from a lumbar spine fusion to stabilize her low back, her injuries also required surgical intervention to set her foot and ankle with pins. I did not personally meet Brittany until months later, when she stepped into my yoga class one Wednesday night. I heard a few of her friends congratulating her for getting back into movement and asking her how her ankle felt during class. I looked down and saw the big scar on her ankle and asked what happened. She said that she had fallen the year before at the gym, and I responded poorly with "Oh that was you."

I recovered quickly after her kind laugh, and we continued to talk about her healing process. She was making a lot of strides but felt incapable of getting back on the climbing wall due to a crippling fear. Climbing had become a vital activity that kept her body, mind, and spirit happy, so the longer she went without climbing, the more isolated she felt from the healing group of friends that she developed at the gym. I explained some of the emotional techniques that I offer and how I felt it could help accelerate her healing. Brittany had never been to a chiropractor and admitted her interest in seeing me was solely for the mentality work, which I was happy to direct care towards. I encourage anyone new to alternative care to trust whatever portal of entry they are comfortable with and set those boundaries early with a new provider. My care should cater to her, not the other way around. When a patient bravely tries chiropractic for the first time, I respect their boundaries but will always use the opportunity to gently educate them about the detailed care that a chiropractor can offer beyond cavitating (popping) joints.

In our first visit, I sensed her anxiety and eased her into the physical aspect of my care, informing her every step of the way what we were doing and why; communication during treatment is key. I found a significant amount of neurological rewiring that needed to be done to improve weak muscles as well as scar tissue that was limiting joint mobility. Her physical progress is a wonderful case, but my purpose in sharing her story is to explain how far someone can fall in life yet still have the strength to rewrite a fear that occupies most of the brain's attention. Beyond helping Brittany find peace with her fall and forgiving the events of that day, her mind-body needed to learn to trust herself again. After trauma, the primitive body is hard to convince that the conscious mind, which controls the surface-level command center, is a worthy captain. It takes some cognitive work to regain deep, soul-level trust after a surgery, accident, or self-injury. The first day Brittany got back on the climbing wall, it had been eight months after her accident.

I greeted her for her fourth visit, inviting her to follow me down the hallway toward my office. I walked in front of her, passing through the fitness room, as I asked my standard question of, "How are you doing today?" She was miles away mentally and disregarded the question. She instead asked, "Has that rock-climbing wall always been there?" We both laughed at how obvious the black wall covered with bright climbing holds was when walking into the fitness room of my office at the time. Prior to that day and that moment, her brain clearly was not ready to acknowledge the wall that she had passed up to eight times previously. At this moment, I knew she was ready to move into a new stage of healing that went beyond the confines of a clinical table.

We worked in baby steps, but I was determined to break the ice that day and help Brittany get back on the wall. Standing at the foot of the wall, we used visualization exercises to remind the brain how shifting her bodyweight would feel. With her feet focused on the supportive ground beneath her, I guided her to select a mental color that represented safety. Brittany responded, "A kind blue, like the color of the walls in the climbing gym's yoga studio." We mentally chalked her hands up with that shade of blue and "painted" the wall and climbing holds in front of her with the color as well. Gently integrating the physical body, I supported her with stools and hands as she tried placing her surgically repaired foot on a tiny foothold. She froze and realized that the color of the route she fell from was a dark blue.

Halting progress, I encouraged her to combine the two shades of blue in her mind's eye so that they would make a new shade, adding some fun variations to make it desirable. Brittany said she added sequins and sparkles to the new color in her mind as we slowly introduced each extremity to the wall to let her new limbs learn what trusting bodyweight felt like. She shook while clinging to the wall but didn't let the heavy breathing deter her from loving her body again. Being a fellow rock climber, I understood her attachment to the sport. It was a beautiful moment to witness her excitement as she inched closer to an important activity that has completely altered her young life. We closed for the day, and both left feeling exhausted yet thankful.

My favorite teaching point with Brittany's story is how important asking for help is and at the right time along the healing journey. I met her at the right time to offer my services—a place along her healing where she was prepared to handle the stress that I would request of her and her body. Having the same introductory conversation a few months before that right moment would have resulted in no action on her part. While committing to change (healing or lifestyle), the journey is not completely up to us. Certain resistances in life need to run their course before the dam opens and allows us to push through. She needed to feel strong and safe on the ground before recognizing a climbing wall was accessible to her new body.

I had the pleasure of climbing several times with Brittany at the climbing gym following the completion of her chiropractic treatment plan. The first time that she scaled to fifty feet on the wall since her fall, we both glowed with pride. In awe of her accomplishment, I sat heavy in my harness to give her time to suspend at the top of the route and process how far she had come. I am very grateful for her trust and will never forget the look on her face as she soaked up the world from such a high vantage point.

I do trust that Brittany would have gotten to this level of change eventually, by herself or with another provider, but not as quickly or as comfortably as we did that day. I genuinely believe that the relationship we create with movement during a healing process should bring ease to the nervous system. Even if you are feeling brave on the surface, if the subconscious mind is revolting out of fear, you're not ready. Healing takes a step backward when putting the nervous system in such distress. Compensatory behavior develops, and unresolved traumas get stored deeply in the body, only to resurface at the next example of pain or injury. Take the time to work through trauma once, so that when you finally come to the starting line, you are fully prepared to work forward.

The Stages of Change

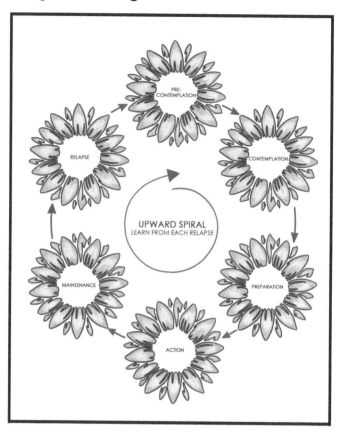

I was first introduced to the transtheoretical model, also called the stages of change model, as an undergraduate student in a health behavior course. The program was developed by James Prochaska in the 1970s to study the mental resistance of a population as they tried to quit smoking. I now use the stages of change model in weekly conversations with patients to help them categorize and organize where along the journey toward change they are feeling stuck. The timeline parameters may not be appropriate for every health behavior or personality type, but I believe the overall theory applies to many resistances in life.

Stage One: Precontemplation

> We must be willing to get rid of
> the life we've planned, so as to
> have the life that is waiting for us.
> — Joseph Campbell, *The Hero with a Thousand Faces*

Prochaska found that in the first stage of making a behavioral change, the subjects had no intention of making a lifestyle change anytime soon (within the next six months). He believed that someone could live in this stage of denial for years if they continue to ignore that a behavior is problematic or negatively affecting their health.[6] This stage represents someone's precontemplation mindset because the state of consciousness at which they are living has yet to rise to a level of awareness where changes are safe to begin contemplating. For most, living in this stage represents "survival mode," where we underestimate the benefits of healthy behavior and are too busy staying above water to entertain the idea of changing a routine. By placing too much emphasis on the risks, we are kept from contemplating how to ignite our first step.

Stage Two: Contemplation

> If a choice supports truth, health,
> happiness, wisdom, and love,
> it's the right choice.
> — Joel and Michelle Levey,
> *Mindfulness, Meditation, and Mind Fitness*

In the second stage of change, those living in denial begin to hear a little voice in their head that urges them to look at life differently. Around every corner, they search for a sign to pacify the feeling that change is coming. Like realizing that you need a haircut, you can't unsee the need for a haircut until you eventually crack and schedule an appointment. Someone living in the contemplation stage recognizes the need to improve a problematic behavior and will weigh the pros and cons of this potential change. The list is important to make, including their perceived barriers and perceived benefits of making the change. Barriers include money, time, lack of support, giving up current comforts, and any other logistical issues that trigger fear. Benefits to making a change include healing, growth, happiness, and a fresh start. Until the perceived benefits outweigh the perceived barriers, those who contemplate will not leap forward and make a change. This stage can last a long time and is suggested to represent someone who plans to blow past self-inflicted limitations within the next six months.

Stage Three: Preparation

> Faith in the endgame helps you live
> through the months or years of buildup.
> — Jim Collins, *Good to Great*

Recognition of a forthcoming change is a crucial step during the contemplation stage, but life cannot proceed toward action without conviction. In the preparation stage, people become determined to commit to themselves and make a change within the next thirty days. Normally small steps at first, they will gather information and plan to apply the preparation while analyzing the influence that it will have on their current lifestyle. This is a messy stage where paranoia and paralyzing doubt are constantly steering the brain back to safety. With each step safely taken, we affirm our own empowering ability to grow closer to the action stage, a place that will benefit from laying the groundwork in this stage.

Preparation is considered the most important stage of change. If skipped or rushed past, Prochaska found that 50 percent of people will relapse within twenty-one days and fall back into contemplation while licking their wounds.[7] After witnessing the efforts of so many patients, I feel confident advising anyone who falls into this category to be careful with seeking excessive advice. We tend to complicate decision-making when conflicting seeds of information bounce around in our head. It is confusing to recall which words belong to our true selves and which have been left over from an external source. Stay in your body, feel what is right, and avoid ruminating any advice that does not match your purpose.

Stage Four: Action

> People who say it cannot be done
> shouldn't interrupt those who are doing it.
> — George Bernard Shaw, Irish playwright

If new behaviors can lead to a healthier life, then it is worth the temporary challenge of finding space for them to manifest. In the fourth stage of change, Prochaska observed subjects who had recently taken a leap of faith and changed their behavior within the last six months. Committing to a temporary adjustment period allowed the lives of his subjects to accept the new routine and cement the change. By learning to apply a lifestyle change, we help our internal and external environments to morph into compatible hosts.

Adjustments will also be made to the original goal of a behavioral change. For example, a patient of mine quit her job to open her own medical practice. Within six months, she was forced to seek a part-time position to cover her finances while her personal practice steadily grew. Instead of viewing this as a failure, she allowed her original mindset to adjust. As she later realized, her healthy change included both jobs and didn't require her to nurture one of them exclusively. If she never allowed herself a time frame for processing life's new direction, she may have quit her personal practice altogether as soon as she surrendered to needing supplemental income. Without a grace period, there is a chance for potential relapse at this stage of transition. Preparing correctly in the previous stages will enable life to unfold during the grace period that you and your loved ones create. Stay strong, ask for help, create an environment that complements the new change, and remember—you've already done the hardest part.

Stage Five: Maintenance

> We must forgive ourselves for
> the errors we made when we were less evolved.
> — David. R Hawkins, *Letting Go*

In this challenging stage, a successfully changed person learns how to sustain their recent growth. A time frame in this stage depends on the specific change made and level of addictive behavior being overcome, but traditionally it extends infinitely past the six-month anniversary of the healthy action taking place. Our journey upward is never over; people in this stage work to prevent relapses or returning to earlier mindsets. Conditioning a new life includes substituting out unhealthy behaviors and thoughts for healthier ones as well as offering ourselves a reward system to reinforce positive behavior. A lot of surprising adjustments naturally take place when you commit to supporting a permanent behavior change. Those who challenge or hinder this new growth start to fade out of the picture to make way for new and supportive recruits. It is extremely challenging to accept when a person or previously enjoyable activity no longer serves the new healthy direction of your life. Without reducing exposure to unhealthy or negatively influencing stimuli, the chance to fall back into relapse is substantial. Self-reevaluation and self-inquiry are both a necessity during this time as we dissect how healthy behavior is in alignment with who we want to become.

Stage Six: Termination

If you want the best that the world has to offer,
offer the world your best.
— Neale Donald Walsch, *Conversations with God*

In the final stage of the behavioral change theory, a successfully changed person has no temptation or desire to undo their hard work or return to the unhealthy version of themselves. Without a relapse, they have built a sense of achievement that paves the way for further progress in other areas of life, usually which complements the initial change that was just made. While momentum is strong, the cycle starts again and will go through its own necessary timeline to carry us all through to the next level of self-progress. Life will not stop offering us chances to learn or grow, so stay patient during your personal journey, and in your own sweet time, move forward.

Remember that the stages of behavioral changes were developed while studying health behavior in a small population of smoking individuals. The numbers and time frames are not an exact science, but when the theories are applied to our current challenges in life, I believe it's an effective organizational template. Creating a timeline for the life span of challenges may be healing but creating a timeline for change is empowering. Accepting that change is imminent is an immensely powerful healing sensation felt by both the subtle mind and physical body. As that agreement surges to the surface, past the filters of fear and resistant excuses, every cell in your body is now on board to create action toward that change.

Willow's Announcement

It's truly only a matter of time before the physical body demands progress if the fearful mind continues to drag its heels. Physical symptoms such as digestive irritation, neck tension, jaw tightness, and low back stress are a few common conditions that I have seen flare up in response to unresolved life transitions. Willow came into my office one winter with sharp neck pain that radiated down into her left wrist. It throbbed and had kept her up each night for the past week. Without any knowledge of how this spontaneous pain started, we ruled out structural misalignments and started releasing spasmed muscles around her throat. In conversation, she discussed how temperamental she had been recently from an overwhelming job and assumed that the emotional roller coaster was contributing to the pain.

We utilized an instrument-assisted soft tissue tool to gently scrape the tight muscles of her jaw until she was close to tears. I stopped working and asked, "Am I pushing too hard?"

"No," she said. "I just realized it's time to tell my boss that I'm quitting my job."

We took a break from manual care as I guided her through meditation. I wanted her to prepare the approach that she felt was needed to express her change and to verbalize how she expected her supervisor to respond. I reminded Willow, "Coming from a place of love, all change should be received well if that person respects your journey and does not feel threatened." She left that session with minimal soreness, but when she returned later that week, she reported being pain-free and, most importantly, emotionally stable. She passionately believed that once she made the phone call to her boss, her lingering symptoms resolved. Deciding to approach change within the safety of your mind is a wonderful tool for preparation but, unfortunately, will only deliver you and your health halfway toward the ultimate destination. The relief that is born from fully implementing change comes from openly sharing an evolving truth with the people who are going to be affected by it the most. They will either be part of its application or part of the motivation that delivered you to that moment. Either way, be brave and broadcast your voice.

Words for Positive Change

The mental dialogue that constantly bombards the subconscious mind will eventually make it to the conscious surface, demonstrating what truly triggers our actions or thoughts. Learning to observe mental self-talk is a developed skill that frees you from a lifetime of oblivious self-sabotage. The same skill can be developed to verbally communicate the sensations felt within the physical or subtle mind-body. The best doctors and yoga teachers have trouble explaining all the sensations we can experience with a man-made language, so instead, we depend on movement and interpretation.

Our communication is limited by the patterns and filters that our brain has developed within society's example. A developing child quickly learns that exasperations without the correct volume or gesture will not produce their desired outcome. Words only have power because we associate them with the power to make a change. To supplement words, we share universal movements to help us understand one another and relay the requests of our internal environments. Combining the skills of mirror neurons, the RAS, and intention understanding with empathy, we can speak the language of anyone we meet.

Throughout my work and this guide, I want to dedicate my life to helping others witness the permanent influence of words that we audibly or inaudibly share as well as the messages we listen to inside our own subconscious conversations. If I can help expose others to what the human body has shown me under the influence of the "right words," no one would take that gift for granted again.

So much knowledge can be obtained from diving deep into the microscopic body, but there is much more to understand about the collective influence of those systems on external sources of life. The imprint of our behavior can live in the cells of other human beings, plants, and animals for centuries. The vibration of words that leave our mouth can influence generations of readers or music lovers far beyond our life span. We have been given a divine ability to observe our conscious thought processes unlike the majority of the species that coinhabit this planet. It is the responsibility then of each healer, scientist, and educator to carefully choose what we share, because words can cut like a knife, build life, and produce every experience in between.

Review Workshop and Questions

1. Organize and clump together the challenges in your life into as few categories as possible.

   a. These are the pillars that need to be revamped (job, relationship, location, community, etc.).

2. Prioritize the order of each pillar from most pressing to least time dependent.

3. For the top change priority, identify which of the stages of change matches your current behavioral outlook, and work on the prompt questions for each stage.

   a. PC. Relate with this stage? Ask yourself who is encouraging the potential future change. If it's not you, chances are you'll stay here for a while. Only when the change comes from a personal desire to self-improve (eventually improving the lives of those around us) can we start the cycle.

   b. C. Make a list of the pros and cons of this change. Be honest and personal. Identify perceived barriers versus threats and answer this for each. Is it that you can't or that you won't?

   c. P. Who are three people you can include while researching potential aid? Asking for help doesn't mean confiding your deepest truths to others, just recognizing a skill set that another person has that can offer a new perspective or opportunity for your growth. Look things up, make the budget, organize your finances, read a good how-to book, and prepare for success.

    d. A. Following in my footsteps, what is one small action step you can take until momentum is built for bigger leaps? In a moment of doubt, remind yourself that the what-ifs deter you from living the what-nows and the what-fors.

    e. M. What are some negative triggers in your current environment that may influence you to backslide? If it's a person who's close to you, what is an approachable way to discuss your needs for the future success of health and happiness?

    f. T. Rejoice, regroup, and celebrate before barreling into a new life transition. Each rewarding triumph is registered in the body for you to easily reference in the next chapter. Use that memory and that sensation for continued encouragement.

"We are the ones we have been waiting for."

EPILOGUE

The Healing Equation:
An Intuitive Provider + An Informed
Patient = An Impetus to Progress

As the provider, in any medical specialty, if you won't take the time to authentically answer a patient's questions or concerns, they will find someone who will. If you miss the opportunity to educate a patient about the status of their condition and the empowering plan for recovery, your patient will find someone else who will. If you refuse to recognize a patient's need to be heard and gently comforted with a rub on their shoulder, they will find someone else with an empathetic heart who will.

Without someone to heal, healing hands cannot elicit their full potential. Don't surrender the vital pillars that make us human to be a businessperson or robotic employee. Push the limits of what traditional health-care offers. Implement your skill sets and teachings in your own life to be an advocate for healthy lifestyle choices, mental dialogue, and interpersonal interactions. Ultimately, be the health-care provider that you would want to go to. There is a rapidly growing population of conscious patients seeking holistic and comprehensive health care. Their needs and intuition are evolving, so it is time for the doctors to upgrade alongside them.

As the patient, or future patient of an alternative care provider, don't be afraid to speak to us. Each question that you ask portrays where you are in your understanding of the body. That level helps your doctor gauge their communication style and ability to make appropriate recommendations. Ask for referrals and resources for further learning at home. Bring your family with you when you visit. Show them what type of care you are seeking and what level of dedication you expect from them to support that healing process once you leave the office. We heal the best when our loved ones heal alongside us, and by exposing our doctor to personal relationship dynamics, the provider will better understand what we are dealing with at home.

To both components of the healing equation, I ask you all to have patience. Healing isn't a quick fix; it's a sustainable progression that adapts to the growing demands of new goals, hobbies, and life challenges. I believe that the most important part of a new patient visit is for both parties to connect on a personal level. Communication that is balanced between humility and conviction allows providers to have the opportunity to offer every skill that they possess. With a wrong first impression, providers may never get the chance to offer an appropriate routine to the people who prefer to heal at home.

Throughout this guide, I've presented sequential chapters of healing insight that you can access in one of two ways; learn the skills yourself or invite a pair of healing hands to perform with you. Trusting the universe to lead you to the right provider is an act of faith, but until the signs all point toward the next level of healing, we are still required to put in the work.

I speak for the entire medical community when I say thank you for teaching us and learning with us.

ACKNOWLEDGMENTS

First and foremost, I am eternally grateful for the loving support of my family. Thank you for taking this journey toward conscious health alongside me. Your willingness to embrace the lifestyle that I was designing made every success possible.

Thank you to the beautiful angels who carried me through life to the next safe stage of personal development. Without your authentic love and patience, I would not have had such a fruitful foundation on which to grow.

Can you be considered a doctor without patients? Thank you to the years of patients who shared their hearts and healing with me. And lastly, to the mentors of my healing hands, thank you for recognizing a passion and guiding me toward that vision. I can't imagine properly repaying you all without paying those gifts forward, so I will dedicate the rest of my learning life toward doing so.

> Go out and do for others what
> somebody did for you.
> — Randy Pausch

ENDNOTES

Chapter 1: Chiropractic Theory

1. Stuart McGill, Low Back Disorders (Champaign, IL: Human Kinetics, 2007), 36.
2. Marco Catani, "Dorsal Column; A Little Man of Some Importance," *Journal of Neurology* 140 (2017): 3055–3061, accessed January 2020.
3. Claudia Anrig, *Pediatric Chiropractic*, 2nd ed. (Wolters Kluwer, 2013), 433–450.
4. Pavel Kolav, *Clinical Rehabilitation* (Rehabilitation Prague School, 2013).
5. Warren Hammer, *Functional Soft-Tissue Examination and Treatment by Manual Methods*, 3rd ed. (Sudbury, MA: Jones and Bartlett Publishers Inc., 2007), 209.
6. Thomas C. Michaud, *Human Locomotion: The Conservative Management of Gait-Related Disorders* (Newton, MA: Newton Biomechanics, 2011), 104.

Chapter 2: Emotional Pain

1. Seaman, David. The Deflame Diet: How to Extinguish Disease-Promoting Inflammation. ACA Publications. 2016. Accessed online 4/2020.
2. O'Connor Annie & Kolski, Melissa. *A World of Hurt: A Guide to Classifying Pain*. Thomas Land Publishers. 2015. Print. Pg. 68

3. Rankin, Lisa. *Mind Over Medicine: Scientific Proof That You Can Heal Yourself.* Hay House Inc. Carlsbad, CA. 2014. Print.

4. Fuchs, Perry. Peng, Yuan Bo. The anterior cingulate cortex and pain processing. Frontiers in Integrative Neuroscience. 2014; 8: 35. Published online 2014 May 5. Accessed Online 4/12/2020.

5. Wickliffe, Abraham et al. Is plasticity of synapses the mechanism of long-term memory storage? NPJ Sci Learn. 2019; 4: 9. Accessed online 2020. May 26.

6. Cosier, Susan. Where Memories Live. SA Mind 26, 3, 14 doi:10.1038/scientificamericanmind0515-14b. Accessed online 3/19/20

Chapter 3: Muscle Testing

1. Anderson, Marcia. Foundations of Athletic Training, 6th Edition. Wolters Kluwer. Online Edition. 2016. Page 100–105.

2. Walther, David. Applied Kinesiology. Systems DC. Pueblo, Colorado. Print. 1988. pg 36, 203–244.

3. Weinstock, David. NeuroKinetic Therapy, an Innovative Approach to Manual Muscle Testing. 2010. Print.

4. Myers, Thomas. *Anatomy Trains.* Churchill Livingstone. New York, NY. 2014. Pgs 184–190. Print.

5. Cook, Gray. *Movement: Functional Movement System.* On Target Publications. Aptos, CA. 2010. Print.

6. Critchley, Hugo. Electrodermal Responses: What Happens in the Brain. *The Neuroscientist.* Volume: 8 issue: 2, page(s): 132–142. 2002. Accessed online 3/30/2020.

7. Omura, Yoshiaki. Basic principles of Bi-digital O-ring test. International Conference on Dentistry and Integrated Medicine. Web. 2018. Accessed online. 3/31/20

Chapter 4: Acupuncture & Becoming A Healer

1. Nelson, Bradley. The Emotion Code. St. Martin's Essentials. New York. 2019. Pg 103. Print.

2. Myers, Thomas. *Anatomy Trains.* Churchill Livingstone. New York, NY. 2014. Pgs 184–190. Print.

3. Langevin HM, Churchill DL, Wu J, et al. Evidence of connective tissue involvement in acupuncture. *FASEB J.* 2002;16(8):872–874. doi:10.1096/fj.01-0925fje. Web Accessed 6/3/2020.

4.   Walther, David. Applied Kinesiology. Systems DC. Pueblo, Colorado. Print. 1988. pg 36, 203–244.

5.   Ahn AC, Park M, Shaw JR, McManus CA, Kaptchuk TJ, Langevin HM. Electrical impedance of acupuncture meridians: the relevance of subcutaneous collagenous bands. *PLoS One*. 2010;5 (7): e11907. Published 2010 Jul 30. doi:10.1371/journal.pone.0011907. Web Accessed 6.4.20.

6.   Nencini S, Ivanusic JJ. The Physiology of Bone Pain. How Much Do We Really Know?. *Front Physiol*. 2016;7:157. Published 2016 Apr 26. doi:10.3389/fphys.2016.00157

Chapter 5: Quantum Healing

1.   Chopra, Deepak. Quantum Healing: Exploring the Frontiers of Mind/Body Medicine. Bantam Books Publishing. Print. 1989. Pgs. 45–50.

2.   Dr. Mamta Patel Nagaraja. *Dark Energy, Dark Matter*. June 19,2020. Web Accessed. 6.19.2020. https:science.nasa.gov/astrophysics/focus-areas/what-is-dark-energy

3.   Ross CL. Energy Medicine: Current Status and Future Perspectives. *Glob Adv Health Med*. 2019;8:2164956119831221. Published 2019 Feb 27. doi:10.1177/2164956119831221

4.   Children, Martin, and Beech, *The HeartMath Solution*. Harper One Publishing. *Print. 2000. p.33.*

5.   Anindita Roy Chowdhury and Anshu Gupta (2015). Effect of Music on Plants – An Overview, International Journal of Integrative Sciences, Innovation and Technology (IJIIT), 4(6), 30–34.

6.   Calamassi. Pomponi. Music Tuned to 440 Hz Versus 432 Hz and the Health Effects: A Double-blind Cross-over Pilot Study. *Explore*. Volume 15, Issue 4. 2019. Pages 283–290. Web Accessed 6.11.2020.

7.   Dispenza, Joe. *Becoming Supernatural. HayHouse Publishing. Carlsbad, CA. 2017. Print. Pages: 61-68.*

8.   Exploring the Role of the Heart in Human Performance: An Overview of Research Conducted by the HeartMath Institute. Science of the Heart: Vol 1 (1993-2001)

9.   Teimori F, Khaki AA, Rajabzadeh A, Roshangar L. The effects of 30 mT electromagnetic fields on hippocampus cells of rats. *Surg Neurol Int*. 2016;7:70. Published 2016 Jun 29. doi:10.4103/2152-7806.185006

Chapter 6: Yoga Philosophy

1. Assaf, AM. Academic stress-induced changes in Th1- and Th2-cytokine response. 2017 Dec;25(8):1237-1247. doi: 10.1016/j.jsps.2017.09.009. Epub 2017 Sep 25. Web.

2. Kiecolt-Glaser, Janice. Stress, Food, and Inflammation: Psychoneuroimmunology and Nutrition at the Cutting Edge. Psychosomatic Med. 2010 May; 72(4): 365–369. Web.

3. Rankin, Lisa. *Mind Over Medicine: Scientific Proof That You Can Heal Yourself.* Hay House Inc. Carlsbad, CA. 2014. Print.

4. Berezin, Robert. *The Secrets of Consciousness, the limbic-cortex is organized as a drama in the brain.* June 2017. Web Accessed 8.25.2020.

5. Howren, M, et al. Associations of Depression with C-reactive Protein, IL-1, and IL-6: a meta-analysis. Psychosom Med. 2009 Feb;71(2):171–86. Epub 2009 Feb 2. Web.

6. Long, Ray. *The Key Poses of Yoga.* Print. Pg. 3–24.

7. *McKenzie Method of Mechanical Diagnosis & Therapy Lumbar Spine.* 2015. Print. Pg. 10

8. O'Connor Annie & Kolski, Melissa. *A World of Hurt: A Guide to Classifying Pain.* Thomas Land Publishers. 2015. Print. Pg. 68

9. Bordini, Bruno. The Continuity of the Body: Hypothesis of Treatment of the Five Diaphragms. *Journal of Alternative and Complementary Medicine.* 21 (4). 2015. Web accessed July 2020.

10. Rosen, Richard. Pranayama: *Beyond the Fundamentals.* Shambhala Publications. Boston, Massachusetts. 2006. Print. Pg 62.

11. Kolav, Pavel. Clinical Rehabilitation. Rehabilitation Prague School. Print. 2013.

Chapter 7: Affirmations and Mental Barriers

1. Mlodinow, Leonard. Subliminal: How Your Unconscious Mind Rules Your Behavior. First Vintage Books Edition. 2013. Print.

2. Garcia-Rill E, Virmani T, Hyde JR, D'Onofrio S, Mahaffey S. Arousal and the control of perception and movement. *Curr Trends Neurol.* 2016;10:53–64. Accessed Online 4/8/2020.

3. Fenster et al. Brain Circuit Dysfunction in Post-traumatic Stress Disorder: From Mouse to Man. *Nature Reviews Neuroscience.* 19, 535-551 (2018).

4. Napper, Paul. Rao, Anthony Rao. The Power of Agency: The 7 Principles to Conquer Obstacles, Make Effective Decisions, and Create a Life on Your Own. St. Martin's Press, March 2019. Print.

5. Acharya, Sourya. Mirror neurons: Enigma of the metaphysical modular brain. J Nat Sci Biol Med. 2012 Jul-Dec; 3(2): 118–124. Accessed online 4/2020.

6. Prochaska, J. O. and W. F. Velicer (in press). "The transtheoretical model of health behavior change." American Journal of Health Promotion.

7. Prochaska, PH.D., James O., John C. Norcross, PH.D., and Carlo C. Diclemente, PH.D. *Changing for Good.* New York, NY: HarperCollins Publishers, 1994. Print.

INDEX

A

acupuncture ix, 46, 55, 60, 74, 76, 77, 78, 79, 80, 81, 82, 83, 84, 85, 86, 88, 89, 90, 91, 92, 93, 94, 128, 146, 168

affirmations 34, 42, 45, 164, 173, 174, 175, 176, 177, 182, 188, 191

applied kinesiology (AK) 59, 60, 70, 84

asana 132, 133, 154, 167

autonomic nervous system 56, 57, 61, 63, 156

B

behavior (see *stages*) 88, 89, 107, 121, 185, 195, 196, 197, 198, 199, 200, 201, 203

breathing 49, 84, 93, 133, 135, 139, 155, 156, 157, 166, 169, 194

C

central nervous system 4, 11, 152, 165, 183

chakras 80, 87, 128, 158, 159, 160, 161, 162, 163, 164, 165, 166, 167, 168, 189

chemical pain 27, 28

Chinese Medicine (TCM) 76, 79, 87, 88, 89, 160, 168
    elements 62, 88, 89, 107, 168
    meridians. *(see* meridians)
    organs 3, 31, 38, 47, 57, 60, 62, 77, 78, 87, 88, 109, 112, 114, 115, 144, 150, 156, 157, 168, 184

chiropractic xi, 1, 2, 3, 4, 5, 6, 7, 8, 10, 11, 12, 14, 15, 16, 17, 19, 21, 24, 27, 28, 31, 36, 37, 38, 39, 46, 53, 54, 56, 57, 58, 59, 74, 75, 81, 83, 91, 93, 94, 98, 100, 114, 118, 123, 125, 128, 134, 135, 137, 146, 155, 158, 168, 188, 189, 193, 195

connection 5, 8, 27, 37, 43, 48,
    50, 61, 63, 79, 83, 91, 94,
    96, 102, 119, 140, 141, 153,
    156, 158, 161, 163, 165,
    180, 183
consciousness 35, 49, 62, 67, 94,
    120, 121, 141, 146, 197
cortisol 33, 34, 87, 145, 146

D

dan tien 87
dark matter 107, 108
diaphragm 155, 156, 157, 158, 159
dry needling 74, 80, 81

E

electromagnetic fields 64, 107,
    108, 109, 111, 213
emotional pain 24, 26, 27, 36, 37,
    40, 41, 46, 48, 49, 87, 119,
    127, 185
The Emotion Code 49, 66, 78

F

fight-or-flight (see stress response)
    56, 144, 184
frequencies 78, 107, 108, 109, 112,
    113, 116, 117, 118, 148
    emotions x, 22, 29, 32, 34,
        35, 37, 38, 40, 43, 46,
        47, 49, 55, 60, 63, 66,
        77, 78, 84, 85, 94, 95,
        120, 121, 136, 139,
        140, 142, 145, 146, 152,
        160, 161, 163, 164, 176,
        184, 187
    music 8, 110, 111, 112, 116,
        163, 204, 213

G

galvanic skin response 63
glands (see chakras) 145, 160, 162

H

holistic 46, 53, 192, 207

I

indicator muscle testing 55, 63,
    68, 69, 70, 71, 79, 84, 85
inflammation 27, 28, 29, 31, 82,
    83, 145, 146, 153
intuitive healer 121, 139, 166

J

joint centration 151

K

Kho cycle 88

L

limbic system 34, 35, 119,
    145, 152

M

Map of Consciousness 120
medical intuitive 121, 122,
    125, 161
meditation 35, 38, 48, 76, 91, 114,
    124, 143, 144, 148, 149, 166,
    185, 192, 197, 202
meridians 60, 76, 77, 78, 79, 80,
    81, 82, 83, 84, 85, 87, 94,
    160, 168
metaphoric pain 41, 42, 43, 45

metaphysical pain 27, 38, 41, 46, 163
mindfulness 38, 96, 121, 197
muscle testing 45, 54, 55, 57, 58, 59, 60, 61, 62, 63, 64, 66, 67, 68, 69, 70, 71, 79, 84, 85, 93, 187
    energetic 27, 55, 60, 62, 63, 76, 77, 78, 80, 84, 87, 88, 92, 93, 94, 107, 108, 111, 115, 116, 125, 127, 140, 158, 159, 163, 164, 169, 178, 180, 190
    manual 5, 11, 24, 29, 31, 32, 38, 43, 45, 46, 48, 54, 55, 58, 59, 60, 71, 75, 79, 87, 94, 97, 99, 138, 166, 202

N

neurons 11, 35, 38, 186, 187, 203, 215
    mirror neurons 186, 187, 203
neuropeptides 37
neuroplasticity 161
nociception 152, 153

O

O-ring test 64, 66
orthopedic muscle testing 57, 70

P

parasympathetic nervous system 48, 56, 153
perception 5, 10, 21, 34, 60, 95, 97, 99, 101, 119, 130, 162, 176, 177, 182, 183, 185, 186, 187, 191

post-traumatic stress disorder 184
pranayama 156
pressure waves 116
psychosomatic pain 27, 32, 35, 39, 151

Q

qi ("chee") 76, 77, 78, 87
qigong 87, 168
quantum 62, 106, 107, 108, 109, 110, 111, 112, 114, 115, 116, 122, 129
    healing ix, x, xiii, 2, 5, 6, 8, 9, 13, 14, 16, 17, 18, 24, 26, 28, 29, 30, 33, 35, 36, 39, 40, 41, 42, 45, 48, 52, 53, 54, 55, 56, 59, 62, 63, 64, 72, 76, 77, 78, 81, 82, 83, 84, 91, 92, 93, 94, 95, 96, 97, 100, 101, 102, 106, 107, 109, 110, 111, 113, 114, 115, 116, 119, 120, 123, 126, 127, 128, 129, 132, 133, 136, 137, 138, 139, 140, 141, 142, 144, 145, 146, 148, 151, 153, 154, 159, 160, 161, 166, 167, 168, 173, 177, 178, 180, 185, 187, 189, 190, 191, 192, 193, 194, 195, 198, 201, 207, 208
    physics 25, 106, 107, 109, 110, 111, 113, 115, 116

R

reality 39, 67, 101, 107, 124, 129, 136, 139, 162, 182, 183, 187

receptors 3, 37, 54, 116, 128, 150,
    152, 153
  joint 2, 3, 4, 5, 8, 10, 12, 16,
      19, 28, 29, 30, 36, 37,
      43, 47, 54, 55, 57, 66,
      81, 83, 85, 89, 110,
      121, 132, 149, 150, 151,
      153, 154, 156, 157, 158,
      166, 193
  neuropeptides 37
  pain. *(see* nociception)
reticular activating system 183,
    185, 186

S

sensory gating 184
stages of behavioral change 201
stress response 35, 144, 145, 146
subtle body 128, 140, 141,
    159, 166
sympathetic nervous system 144,
    145, 153

T

tendinopathy 154
tensegrity 12, 13
Traditional Chinese Medicine
    (TCM) 76, 88, 89

V

vibrations x, 62, 77, 79, 105, 111,
    112, 116, 119, 120, 161, 169,
    174, 177, 178, 203

W

Wolff's law 114

Y

yoga ix, 14, 24, 27, 36, 38, 39,
    40, 49, 53, 55, 68, 80, 87,
    97, 98, 99, 101, 112, 121,
    124, 127, 128, 131, 132,
    133, 134, 135, 136, 137,
    138, 139, 140, 141, 142, 143,
    144, 146, 148, 149, 150, 151,
    152, 153, 154, 155, 156,
    157, 158, 159, 160, 164, 165,
    166, 167, 168, 169, 170, 171,
    173, 179, 189, 192, 194, 203
  mechanics 57, 80, 108, 113,
      126, 151
  mudras 167, 168, 169
  philosophy 7, 27, 39, 56, 60,
      77, 81, 85, 89, 93, 100,
      121, 128, 132, 133,
      142, 156, 159, 160, 164,
      168, 170